LIBRARY
EDUCATION CENTRE
PRINCESS ROYAL HOSPITAL

TELFORD HEALTH LIBRARY
Princess Royal Hospital

01952 641222 ext 4440
telford.library@sath.nhs.uk

TELFORD HEALTH LIBRARY

£19.99
WA 206 CAN
28 Day Loan

KT-148-512

ABC of

Learning and Teaching in Medicine

Second Edition

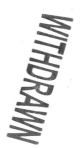

TELFORD

CB015825

ABC series

An outstanding collection of resources - written by specialists for non-specialists

The *ABC series* contains a wealth of indispensable resources for GPs, GP registrars, junior doctors, doctors in training and all those in primary care

- **Now fully revised and updated**

- **Highly illustrated, informative and practical source of knowledge**

- **An easy-to-use resource, covering the symptoms, investigations, treatment and management of conditions presenting in your day-to-day practice and patient support**

- **Full colour photographs and illustrations aid diagnosis and patient understanding of a condition**

For more information on all books in the *ABC series*, including links to further information, references and links to the latest official guidelines, please visit:

www.abcbookseries.com

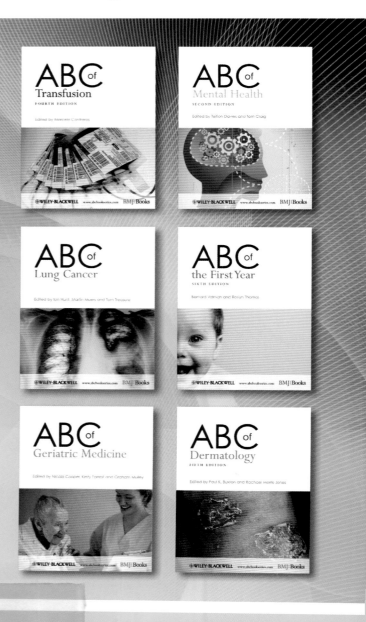

⊕WILEY-BLACKWELL   BMJ|Books

ABC of

Learning and Teaching in Medicine

Second Edition

EDITED BY

Peter Cantillon

Professor
Department of General Practice
National University of Ireland, Galway
Galway, Ireland

Diana Wood

Director of Medical Education and Clinical Dean
University of Cambridge;
School of Clinical Medicine
Addenbrooke's Hospital
Cambridge, UK

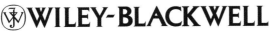
WILEY-BLACKWELL
A John Wiley & Sons, Ltd., Publication

BMJ|Books

This edition first published 2010, © 2010 by Blackwell Publishing Ltd
Previous edition: 2003

BMJ Books is an imprint of BMJ Publishing Group Limited, used under licence by Blackwell Publishing which was acquired by John Wiley & Sons in February 2007. Blackwell's publishing programme has been merged with Wiley's global Scientific, Technical and Medical business to form Wiley-Blackwell.

Registered office: John Wiley & Sons Ltd, The Atrium, Southern Gate, Chichester, West Sussex, PO19 8SQ, UK

Editorial offices: 9600 Garsington Road, Oxford, OX4 2DQ, UK

The Atrium, Southern Gate, Chichester, West Sussex, PO19 8SQ, UK

111 River Street, Hoboken, NJ 07030-5774, USA

For details of our global editorial offices, for customer services and for information about how to apply for permission to reuse the copyright material in this book please see our website at www.wiley.com/wiley-blackwell

The right of the author to be identified as the author of this work has been asserted in accordance with the Copyright, Designs and Patents Act 1988.

All rights reserved. No part of this publication may be reproduced, stored in a retrieval system, or transmitted, in any form or by any means, electronic, mechanical, photocopying, recording or otherwise, except as permitted by the UK Copyright, Designs and Patents Act 1988, without the prior permission of the publisher.

Wiley also publishes its books in a variety of electronic formats. Some content that appears in print may not be available in electronic books.

Designations used by companies to distinguish their products are often claimed as trademarks. All brand names and product names used in this book are trade names, service marks, trademarks or registered trademarks of their respective owners. The publisher is not associated with any product or vendor mentioned in this book. This publication is designed to provide accurate and authoritative information in regard to the subject matter covered. It is sold on the understanding that the publisher is not engaged in rendering professional services. If professional advice or other expert assistance is required, the services of a competent professional should be sought.

The contents of this work are intended to further general scientific research, understanding, and discussion only and are not intended and should not be relied upon as recommending or promoting a specific method, diagnosis, or treatment by physicians for any particular patient. The publisher and the author make no representations or warranties with respect to the accuracy or completeness of the contents of this work and specifically disclaim all warranties, including without limitation any implied warranties of fitness for a particular purpose. In view of ongoing research, equipment modifications, changes in governmental regulations, and the constant flow of information relating to the use of medicines, equipment, and devices, the reader is urged to review and evaluate the information provided in the package insert or instructions for each medicine, equipment, or device for, among other things, any changes in the instructions or indication of usage and for added warnings and precautions. Readers should consult with a specialist where appropriate. The fact that an organization or Website is referred to in this work as a citation and/or a potential source of further information does not mean that the author or the publisher endorses the information the organization or Website may provide or recommendations it may make. Further, readers should be aware that Internet Websites listed in this work may have changed or disappeared between when this work was written and when it is read. No warranty may be created or extended by any promotional statements for this work. Neither the publisher nor the author shall be liable for any damages arising herefrom.

Library of Congress Cataloging-in-Publication Data

ABC of learning and teaching in medicine / edited by Peter Cantillon and Diana Wood. – 2nd ed.
     p. ; cm. – (ABC series)
  Includes bibliographical references and index.
  Summary: "There remains a lack of brief, readily accessible and up to date medical education articles that are of direct use to clinician teachers. Yet their teaching roles are becoming more demanding and there is an increasing expectation that clinician teachers will gradually professionalize what they do. Much has changed in the themes and subjects covered by the original ABC in the past four years. The current edition is effectively out of date particularly in the areas of course design, collaborative learning, small group teaching, feedback, assessment and the creation of learning materials" – Provided by publisher.
  ISBN 978-1-4051-8597-4 (pbk.)
1. Medicine – Study and teaching. I. Cantillon, Peter. II. Wood, Diana. III. Series: ABC series (Malden, Mass.)
  [DNLM: 1. Education, Medical. 2. Teaching – methods. 3. Learning. W 18 A134 2010]
  R735.A65 2010
  610.71 – dc22
                                                                                                2010015123

ISBN: 9781405185974

A catalogue record for this book is available from the British Library.

Set in 9.25/12 Minion by Laserwords Private Limited, Chennai, India
Printed and bound in Malaysia by Vivar Printing Sdn Bhd

1   2010

Contents

Contributors

John Bligh, BSc MA MMEd MD FRCGP Hon FAcadMed

Dean of Medical Education and Professor of Clinical Education
University of Cardiff
Cardiff, UK; *and*
President, Academy of Medical Educators

Julie Brice, BA FAcadMed

Academic Support Manager
Peninsula College of Medicine and Dentistry
Universities of Exeter and Plymouth
Plymouth, UK

Jo Brown, RGN SCM BSc (Hons) MSc PgCAP FHEA

Senior Lecturer in Clinical Communication
St George's, University of London
London, UK

Peter Cantillon, MB BCH BAO MRCGP MSc MHPE

Professor
Department of General Practice
National University of Ireland, Galway
Galway, Ireland

Richard L. Cruess, MD

Professor of Surgery
Member, Center for Medical Education
McGill University
Montreal, Quebec, Canada

Sylvia R. Cruess, MD

Professor of Medicine
Member, Center for Medical Education
McGill University
Montreal, Quebec, Canada

Dason Evans, MBBS MHPE FHEA

Senior Lecturer in Medical Education
St George's, University of London
London, UK

Anne Hesketh, BSc(Hons) Dip Ed

Senior Education Development Officer (now retired)
Postgraduate Medical Office
University of Dundee
Dundee, UK

Eric Holmboe, MD

Chief Medical Officer and Senior Vice President
American Board of Internal Medicine
Philadelphia, Pennsylvania, USA

David Jaques, BSc MPhil Ac Dip Ed

Fellow, Staff and Educational Development Association;
Fellow, Higher Education Academy
London, UK

David M. Kaufman, MEng EdD

Professor, Faculty of Education
Simon Fraser University
Burnaby, British Columbia, Canada

Jean Ker, BSc MD FRCGP FRCPE

Director, Institute of Health Skills and Education
College of Medicine, Dentistry and Nursing
University of Dundee
Dundee, UK

Karen Mann, PhD

Professor, Faculty of Medicine
Dalhousie University
Halifax, Nova Scotia, Canada

Jillian Morrison, PhD FRCP

Professor of General Practice and Head of Undergraduate Medical School
University of Glasgow
Glasgow, UK

John Norcini, PhD

President and CEO
Foundation for Advancement of International Medical Education and Research (FAIMER)
Philadelphia, Pennsylvania, USA

Joan Sargeant, PhD

Associate Professor, Faculty of Medicine
Dalhousie University
Halifax, Nova Scotia, Canada

Lambert W.T. Schuwirth, MD

Professor, Department of Educational Development and Research
Maastricht University
Maastricht, The Netherlands

John Spencer, FRCGP FAcadMedEd

Sub Dean for Primary and Community Care
School of Medical Sciences Education Development
Faculty of Medical Sciences
Newcastle University
Newcastle, UK

Yvonne Steinert, PhD

Associate Dean, Faculty Development;
Director, Centre for Medical Education;
Professor, Department of Family Medicine
Faculty of Medicine
McGill University
Montreal, Quebec, Canada

Jill Thistlethwaite, BSc MBBS PhD MMEd FRCGP FRACGP

Director of the Institute of Clinical Education
Warwick Medical School
University of Warwick
Coventry, UK

Cees P. M. van der Vleuten, PhD

Professor and Chair
Department of Educational Development and Research
Maastricht University
Maastricht, The Netherlands

Val Wass, BSc FRCP FRCGP MHPE PhD FHEA

Head of Keele Medical School
Keele University
Keele, UK

Diana Wood, MA MD FRCP

Director of Medical Education and Clinical Dean
University of Cambridge;
School of Clinical Medicine
Addenbrookes Hospital
Cambridge, UK

Preface

It is 7 years since publication of the first edition of *ABC of Learning and Teaching in Medicine*, during which time much has changed in medical education. Greater recognition of the importance of basing educational design on sound theoretical footings has been accompanied around the world by more direct involvement of governments and regulatory bodies in the organisation and delivery of undergraduate education and postgraduate training. Medical education at all levels has recognised a need to respond to the wider demands of the public, employers and regulatory bodies, to ensure that medical graduates are fit for practice, that junior doctors gain appropriate knowledge and expertise in their chosen field and that specialists are able to develop and adapt in a rapidly changing health-care environment. As a result of these changes, many more doctors have become interested in medical education and have pursued formal training to enhance their abilities as teachers and learners.

Throughout all of this, the basic skills of good medical teachers remain largely unchanged. The original *ABC of Learning and Teaching in Medicine* was conceived as an introductory and accessible text on medical education, illustrating the way in which educational theory and research underpins the practicalities of learning and teaching in medicine. In this second edition, our aim has been to preserve that original aim, whilst introducing some new material including chapters on Medical Professionalism, Faculty Development and Students in Difficulty. Once again, we have invited a group of international authors to contribute and, as editors, we are very grateful to them for their expert contributions. We should like to thank all the staff at Wiley-Blackwell who have been involved in this project and in particular Laura Quigley, Karen Moore and Adam Gilbert.

We hope that readers will find this second edition of the *ABC of Learning and Teaching in Medicine* interesting, stimulating and valuable to them in their daily work.

Diana Wood
Peter Cantillon

LIBRARY
EDUCATION CENTRE
PRINCESS ROYAL HOSPITAL

CHAPTER 1

Applying Educational Theory in Practice

David M. Kaufman

Simon Fraser University, Burnaby, British Columbia, Canada

OVERVIEW

- Medical education has accumulated a useful body of theory that can inform practice
- Three educational theories can be applied in practice: social constructivism, experiential learning and communities of practice (CoPs)
- The range of cognitive skills that can be developed with expert guidance or peer collaboration exceeds what can be attained alone
- Experiential learning is a spiral model with four elements: (i) the learner has a concrete experience; (ii) the learner observes and reflects on this experience; (iii) the learner forms abstract concepts about the experience and (iv) the learner tests the concepts in new situations
- Effective knowledge translation (KT) is dependent on meaningful exchanges among CoP members for information to be used in practice or decision-making

Introduction

When confronted with a challenge in our clinical teaching, wouldn't it be a relief if we could turn to a set of guiding principles based on evidence or long-term successful experience? Fortunately, the field of education has accumulated a useful body of theory that can inform practice. The old adage that 'there is nothing more practical than a good theory' still rings true today. In the first edition of the *ABC of Learning and Teaching in Medicine*, I discussed the application of adult learning theory (andragogy), self-directed learning, self-efficacy, constructivism and reflective practice to the work of medical educators (Kaufman 2003). In this chapter, I extend that discussion by addressing three additional educational theories and show how these could be applied in the context of three case studies; these theories are social constructivism, experiential learning and communities of practice (CoPs). In social constructivism, we are talking about how learners learn from and with peers and in interactions with their tutors. In

experiential learning, we are talking about how learners process and learn from concrete events and experiences. Lastly, in CoPs, we are talking about how learners are socialised into a profession and how they learn through participation in their professional community. Let's examine these three theories in more detail (Overview box).

Social constructivism

The primary idea of constructivism (i.e. cognitive constructivism) is that learners construct their own knowledge based on what they already know, and make judgements about when and how to modify their knowledge. There are some important implications of adopting a constructivist perspective. First, the teacher is not viewed primarily as a transmitter of knowledge but as a guide who facilitates learning. Second, since learning is profoundly influenced by learners' prior knowledge, teachers should provide learning experiences that expose inconsistencies between students' current understandings and their new experiences. Third, teachers should engage students in their learning in an active way, using relevant problems and group interaction. This is not just about keeping learners busy but the interaction must activate students' prior knowledge and lead to the reconstruction of knowledge. Fourth, if new knowledge is to be actively built, sufficient time must be provided for in-depth examination of new experiences.

Vygotsky (1978) elaborated this theory describing 'social constructivism', which posits that learners' understanding and meaning grow out of social encounters. The major theme of Vygotsky's theoretical framework is that social interaction with teachers and other learners plays a fundamental role in the development of understanding. An important aspect of Vygotsky's theory is the idea that cognitive development occurs in a zone of proximal development (ZPD). Vygotsky's (1978) often-quoted definition of ZPD is

... the distance between the actual developmental level as determined by independent problem solving and the level of potential development as determined through problem solving under adult guidance, or in collaboration with more capable peers

– (1978, p. 86)

Full development of the ZPD depends upon full social interaction (Figure 1.1). Vygotsky asserts that the range of cognitive skills that

---

ABC of Learning and Teaching in Medicine, 2nd edition.
Edited by Peter Cantillon and Diana Wood. © 2010 Blackwell Publishing Ltd.

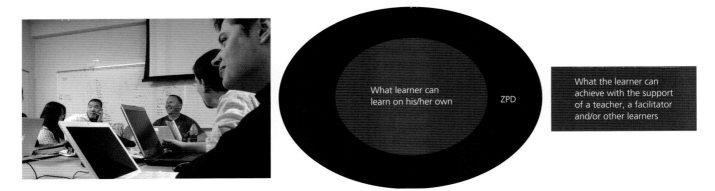

Figure 1.1 Students in a small-group discussion.

can be developed with expert guidance or peer collaboration exceeds what can be attained alone.

The concept of 'scaffolding' is closely related to the ZPD and was developed by other sociocultural theorists applying Vygotsky's ZPD to educational contexts (Wood *et al.* 1976). Scaffolding is a process through which a teacher or more competent peer gives help to the student in her or his ZPD as necessary and then gradually reduces the help as the student becomes more competent. Effective teaching is therefore about identifying the student's current state (prior knowledge) and offering opportunities and challenges that are slightly ahead of the learner's development, i.e. on challenging tasks they could not solve alone. The more able participants (or the experts) model appropriate problem-solving behaviours, present new approaches to the problem and encourage the novice (or the learner) to take on some parts of the task. As novices develop the abilities required, they should receive less assistance and solve more of the problem independently. Simultaneously, of course, they will encounter yet more challenging tasks on which they will continue to receive help (Box 1.1).

Box 1.1 **Social constructivism**

- Learners actively construct their own knowledge, influenced strongly by what they already know.
- Social interaction plays a fundamental role in the development of understanding and meaning.
- The range of cognitive skills developed with expert guidance or peer collaboration exceeds what can be attained alone.
- Effective teaching is slightly ahead of the learner's development, with novices working with more capable others on challenging tasks they could not solve alone.

Experiential learning

Experiential learning theory (Kolb 1984) is a model of learning that posits that learning is a four-step process. It describes how learners learn from experience through four steps: (i) the learner has a concrete experience; (ii) the learner observes and reflects on this experience; (iii) the learner forms abstract concepts about the

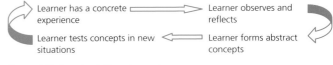

Figure 1.2 Experiential learning cycle.

experience; and (iv) the learner tests the concepts in new situations (Figure 1.2). Kolb asserts that experiential learning can begin at any one of the four steps and that the learner cycles continuously through these four steps. In practice, the learning process often begins with a person carrying out a particular action and then seeing its effect. Following this, the second step in the cycle is to understand these effects in the particular instance to be able to anticipate what would be the result in a similar situation. Following the pattern, the third step would involve understanding the general principle under which the particular instance falls, for example, by looking up the literature or talking to a colleague.

When the general principle is understood, the last step, according to Kolb, is its application through action in a new circumstance. Two aspects can be seen as especially noteworthy: (i) the use of concrete experience to test ideas and (ii) the use of feedback to change practices and theories (Kolb 1984: p. 21–22) (Figure 1.3). Learners along the medical educational continuum use various experiential learning methods such as (i) apprenticeship; (ii) internship or practicum; (iii) mentoring; (iv) clinical

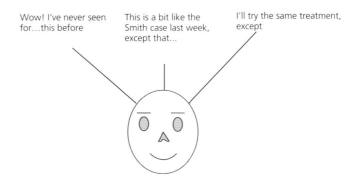
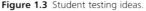

Figure 1.3 Student testing ideas.

supervision; (v) on-the-job training; (vi) clinics and (vii) case study research (Box 1.2).

Box 1.2 **Experiential learning**

- Learning is a four-step cyclical (or spiral) process: feeling, thinking, watching and doing.
- Experiential learning can begin at any of the four steps.
- Each step allows a learner to reflect and form new principles and theories to guide future situations.
- Concrete experience is used to test ideas and these are modified through feedback.

Communities of practice

The term *community of practice* (CoP) was proposed by Lave and Wenger (1991) to capture the importance of integrating individuals within a professional community, and of the community in correcting and/or reinforcing individual practices. For example, a student joining a clinical team for a period of 6 weeks starts as an observer but gradually gets drawn into becoming a participant in team activities and interaction – this is a powerful driver of professional socialisation and the acquisition of professional norms and practices. There are many examples of CoPs including online communities and discussion boards. Barab *et al.* (2002, p. 495) later described a CoP as 'a persistent, sustaining social network of individuals who share and develop an overlapping knowledge base, set of beliefs, values, history and experiences focused on a common practice and/or mutual enterprise.' Within this context, learning can be conceived as a path in which learners move from *legitimate peripheral participant* (e.g. observer, questioner) to core participant of the CoP.

CoPs have gained prominence primarily as vehicles for KT, which refers to the acceleration of the process of making the most current information available for use. Effective KT is dependent on meaningful exchanges among network members for using the most timely and relevant evidence-based, or experience-based, information for practice or decision-making. CoPs are natural places for partnerships and exchanges to start and grow; in them, relevant learning occurs when participants raise questions or perceive a need for new knowledge. Moreover, internet technologies enable these discussions to occur in a timely manner among participants regardless of physical location and time zone, with discussions archived for review at a later date or by those who miss a discussion (Box 1.3).

There are a number of key factors that influence the development, functioning and maintenance of CoPs. The initial CoP membership is important. For example, a medical team with undergraduate and postgraduate students and a clinical mentor would be a typical and legitimate CoP. The commitment to the CoP goals, its relevance and members' enthusiasm about the potential of the CoP to have an impact on practice are also key success factors. On the practical side, a strong infrastructure and resources are essential attributes; these include good information technology,

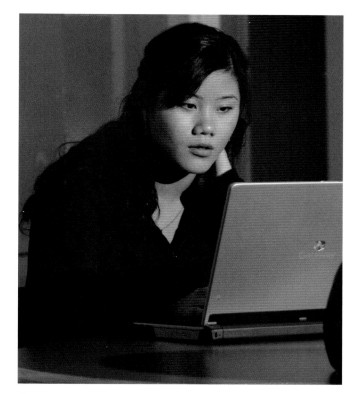

Figure 1.4 Student participating in an online CoP.

useful library resources, databases and human support. In order to provide these key factors, one or more strong, committed and flexible leaders are needed to help guide the natural evolution of the CoP (Figure 1.4).

Box 1.3 **Communities of practice**

- A CoP is a persistent, sustaining social network of individuals who share and develop an overlapping knowledge base, and focus on a common practice and/or mutual enterprise.
- Within this context, learning can be conceived as a path in which learners move from 'legitimate peripheral participant' to core participant of the CoP.
- CoPs have gained their prominence primarily as vehicles for *knowledge translation*, which depends on meaningful exchanges among network members.
- Internet technologies enable discussions to occur in a timely manner among participants regardless of physical location and time zone, with the discussions archived.

Implications for medical educators

In this chapter, three educational theories have been presented, each of which can guide our teaching practices. Some theories will be more helpful than others in particular contexts. However, a number of principles also emerge from these theories, and these can provide helpful guidance for medical educators (Box 1.4).

Box 1.4 **Eight principles to guide educational practice**

1. Learning is an active, rather than a passive mental process, with learners making judgements about when and how to modify their knowledge.
2. Learners should be given opportunities to develop their own understanding through self-directed learning, combined with dialogue with their teachers and peers.
3. Learners should be given some challenging tasks they could not solve independently, and then work on these with more capable others (teachers or peers); as they develop the abilities required, they should receive less assistance and work more independently.
4. Learning should be closely related to the understanding and solution of real-world problems.
5. Learners should complete the full experiential learning cycle in order to gain a complete understanding of a concept; the steps in the cycle are concrete experience, observation and reflection, forming abstract concepts and testing the concepts in new situations.
6. Learners should be given opportunities and support for practice, accompanied by self-assessment and constructive feedback from their teachers and peers.
7. Learners should be given opportunities to reflect on their practice, through analysing and critiquing their own performance and, consequently, developing new perspectives and options.
8. Learners should be included in a CoP focused on a clinical specialty, involving their peers, more senior learners, clerks, registrars, clinicians and others. The CoP will support meaningful exchanges among network members about the most timely and relevant evidence-based, or experience-based, information for practice or decision-making.

Back to the 'real-world' situations

How do the three educational theories described here, and the principles that emerge from them, guide us in the three cases presented? (Box 1.5)

Case 1. You would prepare an interactive lecture on the autonomic nervous system (principle 1), and include a clinical example of its application (principle 4). By interactive, I mean a lecture in which you would plan to stop at key points and interact with the students. A note-taking guide would be distributed in advance (for students to print from a website) containing key points, space for written notes and two key short answer questions to answer or partially completed diagrams for students to complete before the lecture, requiring higher level thinking and strategically situated in your lecture sequence (principles 1 through 5). You would stop twice while delivering the lecture and ask students to discuss their response to each question with their neighbours (principles 1 through 6). A show of hands would determine the class responses to the question (checking for understanding) and the correct answer then would be given (principles 5 and 6). Finally, you would assign a more challenging learning issue for out-of-class research (principles 1 through 6) and the solution given in a later lecture or posted on the website (principles 5 and 6).

Case 2. You could first invite the registrar to observe you with patients, and do a quick debrief while walking from patient

Box 1.5 **Three cases**

Case 1 – Teaching basic science

You have been asked to give a lecture to the first-year medical class of 120 students on the topic of the autonomic nervous system. This has traditionally been a difficult subject for the class, particularly as it has not been covered by faculty in the problem-based Anatomy course. You wonder how you can make this topic understandable to the class in a single lecture.

Case 2 – Internal medicine training

You are the trainer for a first-year registrar in an Internal Medicine training programme. Your practice is so busy that you have very limited time to spend with her.

You wonder how you can contribute to providing a valuable learning experience for your trainee.

Case 3 – Clerkship academic half-day

You are a member of a course committee in the department of family medicine, which is charged with the task of integrating a weekly academic half-day into the third-year, 12-week, family medicine rotation. However, the students are geographically distributed in clinics and physicians' offices across the region. You wonder how your committee can overcome this obstacle.

to patient, and then at the end of the day (principles 1, 2, 4, 5). To complement this, you would assign a number of appropriate case-based simulations, either online or on CD) for her to work through (principles 1 through 7). There is a strong correlation between experiential learning and simulations. In fact, Kolb described simulations and games as presenting learners with a broad experiential learning environment that offers learners support for active experimentation (Kolb 1984). With your help, the registrar would then develop his or her own learning goals, based on the certification requirements and perceived areas of weakness (principles 1 and 7). These goals would provide the framework for assessing the registrar's performance with patients (principles 6 and 7). You would observe and provide feedback (principles 4 through 7), and the registrar would begin to see patients alone (principles 1 through 7). The registrar would keep a journal (written or electronic) in which he would record the results of each step of the experiential learning cycle: concrete experience, observation and reflection, concepts and/or principles learnt and results of testing in new situations (principles 5 through 7). The registrar would also record in his journal the personal learning issues arising from his patients, would conduct self-directed learning on these (principles 1, 2, 7) and would document his or her findings in the journal (principles 5 through 7). The trainer would provide feedback on the journal (principle 7). If practical, the cohort of registrars would communicate via the internet to discuss their insights and experiences (principle 8).

Case 3. You could meet with your IT department to discuss your needs, and agree either to purchase or develop a CoP software platform. You would enlist your willing departmental colleagues and support staff, and your registrars, to help you design the CoP structure (e.g. table of contents), enrol in the CoP and upload some

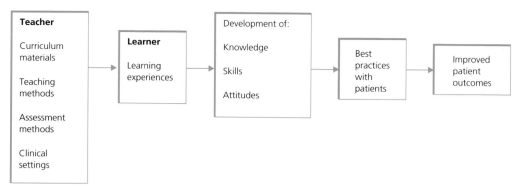

Figure 1.5 The medical education cycle.

content, for example, guidelines, cases, policies, administrative items, website links and so on (principles 1, 2, 8). You would collaborate with the director of the family medicine rotation, and the students would be enrolled in the CoP and assigned the task of uploading some content of their choice as a requirement of the rotation (principles 1, 2, 3, 8). Finally, you would set a schedule for asynchronous case discussions to occur throughout the rotation, with each student having a turn to organise and facilitate the online discussion (principles 1 through 8). These discussions would be archived so that you could provide feedback and a grade at the end of the rotation using a rubric for online discussions (principle 6; see http://www.winona.edu/AIR/rubrics.htm).

Conclusions

This chapter has discussed how to bridge the gap between educational theory and practice. In some situations, a theory can serve as a guide for decisions on educational practice. In other cases, the theory can be used to validate a practice(s) that a medical educator has shown to be effective. In either case, by using teaching and learning methods based on educational theories and derived principles, medical educators can become more effective teachers. This will enhance the development of knowledge, skills and positive attitudes in their learners, and also improve the next generation of teachers. Ultimately, this should result in better trained doctors who provide an even higher level of patient care and improve the outcomes of their patients (Figure 1.5).

Further reading

Kaufman DM, Mann KV. *Teaching and Learning in Medical Education: How Theory Can Inform Practice*. 2nd ed. [Monograph]. London, England: Association for the Study of Medical Education (ASME), 2007.

References

Barab SA, Barnett MG, Squire K. Building a community of teachers: Navigating the essential tensions in practice. *The Journal of the Learning Sciences* 2002; 11(4):489–542.

Kaufman DM. Applying educational theory in practice: ABC of learning and teaching in medicine. *British Medical Journal* 2003;326:213–216. http://www.bmj.com/cgi/content/extract/326/7382/213

Kolb DA. *Experiential Learning*. Englewood Cliffs, NJ: Prentice Hall, 1984.

Lave J, Wenger E. *Situated Learning: Legitimate Peripheral Participation*. Cambridge, UK: Cambridge University Press, 1991.

Vygotsky LS. *Mind in Society: The Development of Higher Psychological Processes*. Cambridge, MA: Harvard University Press, 1978.

Wood D, Bruner J, Ross G. The role of tutoring in problem solving. *Journal of Child Psychology and Psychiatry* 1976;17:89–100.

LIBRARY
EDUCATION CENTRE
PRINCESS ROYAL HOSPITAL

CHAPTER 2

Course Design

John Bligh[1] and Julie Brice[2]

[1]University of Cardiff, Cardiff, UK
[2]Universities of Exeter and Plymouth, Plymouth, UK

OVERVIEW

- Teaching and learning should be enjoyable experiences
- Effective design underpins all successful and enjoyable courses
- Most medical teachers will be involved in course design at some stage
- A five-step approach keeps planning simple and straightforward
- Evaluation of the outcomes of the course is an integral part of high-quality teaching

---

Course design

Teaching, training, appraising and assessing doctors and students are important for the care of patients now and in the future. You should be willing to contribute to these activities.

– *Good Medical Practice*, General Medical Council (2006)

Almost all doctors expect to be involved in teaching during their careers. They are usually engaged in teaching, supervising, examining, appraising and mentoring doctors in training, and many are also involved in teaching undergraduate medical students. A significant number of doctors also engage in teaching colleagues from multi-professional backgrounds. Increasingly, medical students and early career doctors are expected to teach, and many learn the basic skills of a good teacher during their undergraduate years.

While most teachers teach on courses designed by others, an increasing number are becoming involved in course design in their own right or as part of a curriculum or programme team. Designing a course can be a daunting prospect for anyone, but the basic procedure is always the same. We recommend breaking the process down into a simple five-step approach through which the inevitable complexity can be kept under control and a course that can be enjoyable and effective for everyone involved can be produced. The same approach can also be used to plan a programme or a whole curriculum. It is, of course, an iterative process. You may have to go through the steps, in order, more than once before your course is ready for delivery; and as you refine and develop it with feedback,

you will continue to go back to first principles from time to time. But having a basic template will allow you to keep control of the design and preparation of your course so that when you come to deliver it, and subject it to review, you can feel confident that you have considered it from all angles (Box 2.1).

Box 2.1 **Effective course design: the five-step approach**

Step 1: Identify the principles that will underpin your course and define the choices you make.

Step 2: Identify the teaching, learning and assessment processes you will use.

Step 3: Plan and develop the organisational elements that will be required to deliver your course effectively and efficiently.

Step 4: Identify the scope, relevance and timing of the content for each element of your course.

Step 5: Identify the overarching outcomes of your course and decide how it will be evaluated for its overall effect.

Step 1: Identify the principles that will underpin your course and define the choices you make

Designing a course involves making difficult choices about what you will teach, how you will teach it and what you hope will be the results of your teaching. It is much easier to make those choices if you have first thought carefully about the principles and values that underpin your teaching. Every time you come into contact with a student, you are imparting more than just information; you are consciously and unconsciously role modelling a whole set of professional, institutional and personal values, so it is worth taking time to reflect on what these are. Frameworks of curriculum principles have been described, which can be helpful in enabling you to conceptualise what your teaching strategy should be (Box 2.2).

However, in this chapter, we would like to suggest a set of quality principles that reflect current thinking on how medical education should be delivered in order to prepare students optimally for modern clinical practice. They can be summed up in the acronym RIFLE, which stands for Realistic, Integrated, Feedback, Learning and Evaluation (Box 2.3).

Realistic: The most effective medical education takes place where learners can see that what they are learning is of value in terms of its relevance to patient care. Increasing use of real world settings

ABC of Learning and Teaching in Medicine, 2nd edition.
Edited by Peter Cantillon and Diana Wood. © 2010 Blackwell Publishing Ltd.

Box 2.2 **Two key frameworks of curriculum principles**

1. *The PRISMS framework*

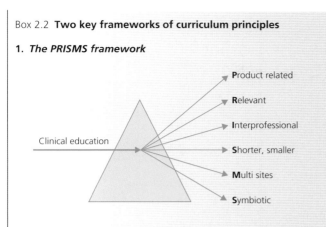

Clinical education

- **P**roduct related
- **R**elevant
- **I**nterprofessional
- **S**horter, smaller
- **M**ulti sites
- **S**ymbiotic

2. *The SPICES model*

SPICES curriculum	Traditional curriculum
Student centred	Teacher centred
Problem based	Information oriented
Interprofessional	Discipline based
Community based	Hospital based
Elective	Uniform
Systematic	Apprenticeship

Data reproduced from Bligh J, Prideaux D, Parsell G. PRISMS: new educational strategies for medical education. *Medical Education* 2001;35:520–521; and Harden RM, Sowden S, Dunn WR. Educational strategies in curriculum development: the SPICES model. *Medical Education* 1984;18:284–297; with permission from Blackwell Publishing Ltd.

Box 2.3 **The RIFLE framework of quality principles for course design**

Realistic
Integrated
Feedback
Learning
Evaluation

---

and materials drawn directly from clinical practice characterise contemporary approaches to course design. Good courses are authentic in terms of the teaching context, the material taught and the resources and teaching materials supplied, and they make use of assessment methods that are directly related to the contexts in which the learners will subsequently be using their learning. Assessment methods are also emerging that simulate reality, such as the integrated structured clinical examination (ISCE), or are based in actual practice, for example, the mini-clinical evaluation exercise (mini-CEX) or direct observation of procedural skills (DOPS).

Integrated: Learners learn best when the information they are acquiring is easily slotted into their existing knowledge frameworks and reinforced and integrated rather than delivered as chunks of disparate or isolated information (the so-called 'string of pearls' approach, where one unrelated course follows another). The best undergraduate courses present material from a variety of disciplines

in an integrated way; deliver basic science teaching that cross-cuts with and informs clinical practice; and, wherever possible, integrate classroom and bedside learning with community teaching. Integrating disciplines, materials, settings and activities will ensure that learners have plenty of opportunity to see how all the elements reinforce and support each other. Careful signposting is important to guide the learner nevertheless.

Feedback: Learners who do not receive adequate, timely and relevant feedback can rapidly become disheartened. Regular feedback is important for maintaining a learner's motivation by reinforcing good performance. It can also reduce anxiety by encouraging him or her to understand and reflect constructively on areas for improvement and growth. A good course ensures that regular feedback opportunities are built in, so that both teachers and learners come to expect and plan for them (Box 2.4). Learners like to compare themselves with their peers too, so opportunities for comparison (but not necessarily competition) should be available.

Box 2.4 **Nicol and Macfarlane-Dick's seven key principles of feedback**

Good feedback

1. helps clarify what good performance is (goals, criteria, expected standards);
2. facilitates the development of self-assessment (reflection) in learning;
3. delivers high-quality information to students about their learning;
4. encourages teacher and peer dialogue around learning;
5. encourages positive motivational beliefs and self-esteem;
6. provides opportunities to close the gap between current and desired performance;
7. provides information to teachers that can be used to help shape teaching.

From: Nicol DJ, Macfarlane-Dick D. Formative assessment and self-regulated learning: a model and seven principles of good feedback practice. *Studies in Higher Education* 2006;31:199–218.

Learning: It may seem obvious that designing a course is all about trainees' learning, and yet many courses are not as successful as they could be because the designers have not laid sufficient emphasis on what and how learners are expected to learn. For example, most students will sit passively if they are required to; but they will enjoy the experience and learn more effectively if they have opportunities to interact, participate, ask questions and take shared responsibility for their own learning experience. Certain types of delivery are more effective depending on the nature, type and number of the learners, the context in which the learning takes place and the material to be learnt. A course design which focuses on how the learners actually learn will ultimately respond better to their needs (Box 2.5).

Personally, I'm always ready to learn, although I do not always like being taught.

– Winston Churchill 1874–1965

Box 2.5 Indicators used in evaluating educational innovations

Structural evaluation measures

- Attendance at class
- Number of applications to medical schools
- Assessment by national body

Outcome evaluation measures

- Career choice or preference
- Nature of practice
- Quality of care indicators
- Student achievement compared with other schools and national norms
- Cost-effectiveness measure
- Effects of different curriculum tracks on assessment and career choice
- Patient satisfaction
- Peer assessment
- Quality of care

Process evaluation

- Group work characteristics (such as tutor and student styles)
- Entry and selection policies
- Assessment practices
- Psychometric measures including learning styles, stress, and so on
- Student satisfaction with medical school

Evaluation tools

- Questionnaires
- Focus groups
- Objective structure clinical examination
- Multiple choice questions
- Viva
- Thesis project
- Qualitative written assessment
- Patient assessment
- Allied health-care professionals' assessment
- Peer evaluation
- Self-assessment

From: Wilkes M, Bligh J. Evaluating educational interventions. *BMJ* 1999;318: 1269–1272.

Box 2.6 Scholarship in teaching: four stages from teaching to research

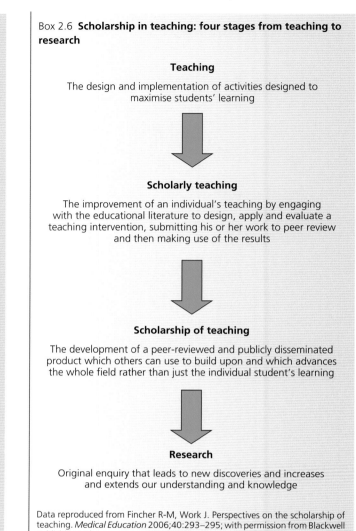

Teaching

The design and implementation of activities designed to maximise students' learning

Scholarly teaching

The improvement of an individual's teaching by engaging with the educational literature to design, apply and evaluate a teaching intervention, submitting his or her work to peer review and then making use of the results

Scholarship of teaching

The development of a peer-reviewed and publicly disseminated product which others can use to build upon and which advances the whole field rather than just the individual student's learning

Research

Original enquiry that leads to new discoveries and increases and extends our understanding and knowledge

Data reproduced from Fincher R-M, Work J. Perspectives on the scholarship of teaching. *Medical Education* 2006;40:293–295; with permission from Blackwell Publishing Ltd.

Evaluation: It is a professional and ethical responsibility of all doctors to improve the quality of care and so medical teachers should be committed to improving clinical care by excellence in teaching. Evaluation is a key element in quality improvement of medical education. Good teachers seek feedback on their own practice and reflect on it so that they can develop their skills, improve their practice and, importantly, demonstrate in a practical way their respect for learners and their colleagues, and their willingness to account for their performance to others. Such 'scholarly' teaching is a hallmark of quality (Box 2.6).

Step 2: Identify the overarching outcomes of your course and decide how it will be evaluated for its overall effect

There may, of course, be several formal ways in which your course will be evaluated, including, in some high-stakes courses, the final grades of your trainees; or feedback from standard-setters, regulators or external examiners; or standardised trainee satisfaction surveys set by the programme managers (Box 2.5). But even where evaluation processes are informal or optional, a good course designer will take care to ensure that students and colleagues have the chance to contribute to the quality improvement process by actively seeking their comments and feedback, reflecting carefully on the information gathered and implementing changes and improvements based on the best available evidence. This is scholarly teaching in action.

Step 3: Identify the teaching, learning and assessment processes you will use

It should be clear to you from your work in Step 1 that your choice of teaching, learning and assessment processes needs to be informed by the best possible educational principles, such as the RIFLE quality framework outlined above. Once you have spent time thinking about your educational principles, identifying effective teaching, learning and assessment strategies becomes easier. Rather than falling back on what has always been done or what is merely convenient, this is now your opportunity to think creatively about how you can maximise the educational opportunities for your students and develop innovative, evidence-based ways of engaging them in their own learning.

> *If the unexamined life is not worth living, the unexamined profession is not worth practising.*
>
> – Edmund D Pellegrino

Your course is likely to be part of a curriculum or programme of study; so to get a clear idea of where your particular element fits in and what the expectations are surrounding your part of the programme, you may need to talk to those who planned it. If you have a well-defined education strategy, it will be easier to demonstrate how the teaching, learning and assessment elements of your course will fit together and enable you to explain and justify your choices clearly to others.

Step 4: Identify the scope, relevance and timing of the content for each element of your course

As Kogan and Shea (2007) observe, medical education differs from most other higher education activities in four key areas.

1 It involves teaching in the clinical setting, which may involve a variety of locations including hospitals, clinics and the community.
2 There are likely to be a much greater number of facilitators involved in delivering aspects of the course, so co-ordination with the overall programme is crucial.
3 Despite the General Medical Council's emphasis on enabling students to select components of the medical curriculum, learners may still find that they are expected to move through their education as a cohort, meaning that the pace of the course may be a problem for some.
4 The structure of the courses within the larger curriculum means that issues such as the overarching organisation of the curriculum, the logicality of the order in which topics are delivered and the need to avoid unnecessary repetition and redundancy are a particular challenge.

Medical teachers need to be especially aware of these issues and ensure that their courses are carefully planned in order to deliver the appropriate material in the most meaningful way at the right time for the learners.

It is important to emphasise that this step (Step 4) in particular is best done as part of a team, and if you wish to make your course truly integrated – as in the RIFLE model – it will actually be impossible to do it otherwise. There are various frameworks that you can use to help you consult with colleagues, subject experts, learners and patients to ensure that your content is appropriate, relevant and timely, such as nominal group technique and the Delphi process.

Step 5: Plan and develop the organisational elements that will be required to deliver your course effectively and efficiently

It is unwise to underestimate the importance of careful management of the organisational aspects of your course. Difficulties with timetabling, accommodation, administration and technology can seriously interfere with teaching and learning and these aspects therefore need careful planning beforehand. You will almost certainly be delivering your course through a hospital, in a general practice setting or in a higher education institution, which may place budgetary, time or physical constraints on the learning opportunities you can provide. What facilities and resources are available? How will quality be ensured and who will evaluate the course? What are the essential requirements and expectations of students and managers, and which can be negotiated? Whom do you need to talk to about this? The list may include colleagues, administrators and finance directors, trainees, managers, patients, carers and the public, international experts and educationists.

Conclusion

Course design is a complex process, but it can be simplified if broken down into five steps. These steps are interrelated and may be revisited more than once, but if you take them in order it will be easier to design and deliver a course that is enjoyable and educationally effective for learner and teacher alike. First, lay the groundwork by identifying the core educational principles of your course. Second, think carefully about what your overall aims are in delivering the course, and consider how they will be evaluated. Third, consider the teaching, learning and assessment processes you will use. Fourth, as part of a team, consult to identify the scope, relevance and timing of the content for each element of your course. Fifth, make certain that the organisational aspects of your course will run smoothly. In this way, you will be building into your course planning a process of continuous quality improvement that is the hallmark of scholarly teaching.

Further reading

Bligh J, Brice J. Further insights into the roles of the medical educator: the importance of scholarly management. *Academic Medicine* 2009;84(8): 1161–1165.

Bligh J, Prideaux D, Parsell G. PRISMS: new educational strategies for medical education. *Medical Education* 2001;35:520–521.

Corrigan O, Ellis K, Bleakley A, Brice J. *Understanding Medical Education: Quality*. Edinburgh: Association for the Study of Medical Education, 2010.

Dent J, Harden RM. *A Practical Guide for Medical Teachers*. London: Churchill Livingstone, 2009.

Kaufman DM, Mann KV. *Understanding Medical Education: Teaching and Learning in Medical Education: How Theory Can Inform Practice*. Edinburgh: Association for the Study of Medical Education, 2007.

Reference

General Medical Council. *Good Medical Practice*. London: General Medical Council, 2006.

Kogan JR, Shea JA. Course evaluation in medical education. *Teaching and Teacher Education* 2007;23:251–264.

CHAPTER 3

Collaborative Learning

Diana Wood

University of Cambridge, Cambridge, UK

OVERVIEW

- Collaborative learning is student centred and promotes active learning
- In medical education the term *Collaborative learning* encompasses a range of small-group learning methods
- Group learning facilitates not only the acquisition of knowledge but also several other desirable attributes, such as communication skills, teamwork, problem-solving, independent responsibility for learning, sharing information and respect for others
- Teachers must encourage student participation while moving towards the educational outcomes
- Staff development is essential to ensure that teachers have the relevant skills as facilitators of collaborative learning

In the wider educational field, the term *collaborative learning* has been applied to a number of different learning methodologies. Broadly speaking, collaborative learning can be thought of as a situation in which two or more people come together to learn – it is student centred and promotes active learning. In medical education, collaborative learning may be regarded as a term which includes a range of teaching and learning techniques generally encompassing small-group work and learning from each other. Group learning facilitates not only the acquisition of knowledge but also several other desirable attributes, such as communication skills, teamwork, problem-solving, independent responsibility for learning, sharing information and respect for others. Acquired at an early stage, the generic skills associated with active, collaborative learning in small groups are of immense value for students moving forward into postgraduate and continuing education and in their clinical careers (Box 3.1 and Figure 3.1).

Discussion groups

Discussion forms the backbone of all active learning techniques, be it teacher-led, student-led or as part of the feedback and reflection process. In its simplest form, discussion allows learners to participate by talking to the teacher and to each other during a teaching session. In reality, the teacher must be well-prepared, willing to listen and to encourage participation. For the novice teacher, this may appear to effect loss of control of the teaching activity. The skill is to encourage student participation by use of appropriate small-group teaching methods while maintaining overall focus towards achievement of the learning goals for the session. Possible roles of the teacher in a discussion group are shown in Box 3.2.

> **Box 3.1 Generic skills and attitudes gained by collaborative learning**
>
> - Teamwork
> - Listening
> - Interpretation of data
> - Explanation of concepts
> - Presentation skills
> - Recording information
> - Cooperation with others
> - Respect for colleagues' views
> - Critical evaluation of literature

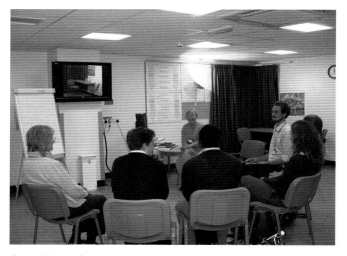

Figure 3.1 Small-group session.

ABC of Learning and Teaching in Medicine, 2nd edition.
Edited by Peter Cantillon and Diana Wood. © 2010 Blackwell Publishing Ltd.

LIBRARY
EDUCATION CENTRE
PRINCESS ROYAL HOSPITAL

Box 3.2 **Possible teacher roles in collaborative learning groups**

- Chairperson
- Facilitator
- Moderator
- Subject expert
- Manager of the learning environment
- Listener
- Referee
- Summarizer

For collaborative learning, teachers must be prepared to accept the risk of uncertainty in the teaching session. When properly prepared, this usually enhances the experience and leads to higher satisfaction amongst teaching staff. In an individual institution, staff development programmes to provide teachers with the skills required to promote active and collaborative learning are essential (Box 3.3).

Box 3.3 **Facilitating a discussion group**

Background	Understand the place of the teaching session in the curriculum
	Know the stage and level of the students
Learning environment	Arrange the room appropriately
	Introductions – ensure that the students know each other and you
	Describe your goals for the session
	Be explicit – explain your wish for participation
	Be supportive throughout – show praise, approval and interest
Set the scene	Present the topic
	Reflect on previous work
	Introduce the task for the current session
Get started	Present a short task for students to consider in pairs/smaller groups before presenting them to the group as a whole
	Ask students to present any written work they have prepared
Involve the students	Ask a student to lead the discussion on a particular topic
	Encourage students to present diagrams, sketches, etc
Ask effective questions	'Why does that happen?'
	'What do you think about?'
	'Can you explain this?'
Be alert to group dynamics	Ensure the participation of all the group members and deal with dominant, non-participant or disruptive students appropriately
Closure	Review the session
	Describe the conclusions
	Link to the faculty goals for the session
	Give advice about the next session

Problems that can arise when running a discussion group may be experienced in other forms of collaborative learning. These include the following:

- The dominant student
- The shy, quiet student
- The non-participant student
- The joker or disruptive student
- Discussion moves away from the topic

Managing group dynamics to promote collaborative learning requires a particular set of skills which should be addressed in staff development programmes, preferably using experiential methods. The teacher must be alert to the needs of all students in a group and be prepared to intervene if the situation develops to the detriment of the learning opportunities. In general, a positive intervention in which the teacher remains encouraging, offering ways to move the discussion on towards the identified goals of the session should be made. Attempts to silence a dominant student harshly or bring in a quiet student abruptly usually only succeed in making a bad situation worse (Figure 3.2).

A student or small group of students who monopolise the discussion affect the learning of the whole group. An appropriately timed intervention may be needed – it is important to balance the needs of the group against the possibility of demotivating enthusiastic participants. Many problems can be avoided by spending some time at the start of a session or group of sessions by discussing the importance of group participation, enabling development of the generic skills associated with collaborative learning. If time and resources permit, the use of video material to illustrate group work can be extremely effective in promoting participation and collaboration in the members of a group.

During the session, it may be necessary to intervene by acknowledging the contributions of dominant members and by deliberately seeking the views of other members of the group. Similar techniques can be used to encourage participation by students who appear uninterested or bored. It may be necessary to meet with these students at the end of a session to identify reasons for non-participation – often lack of preparation or fear of appearing

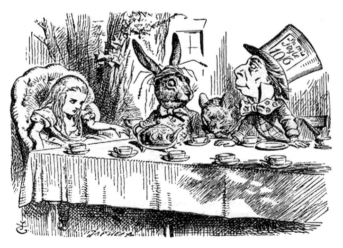

Figure 3.2 A dysfunctional group – a dominant character may make it difficult for other students to be heard.

ignorant may lie behind their behaviour and steps can be taken to address these issues before the next session. The joker or disruptive student can cause particular problems for collaborative learning groups. Often this can be dealt with easily, acknowledging the student's input and reminding him or her of the task in hand. However, again it may be necessary to identify the underlying causes for this behaviour and to draw the student's attention to the effects he or she may be having on the colleagues' learning.

Students value the presence of an expert tutor. If the teacher becomes aware that the discussion is veering away from the topic of the session then it is reasonable to intervene to move things back towards the required subject. This is best achieved by the use of appropriate summarising followed by setting new questions.

Where time and facilities permit, the use of video recording to illustrate group dynamics is of great value. This can provide powerful evidence to the students of the importance of the generic skills required for and learnt by effective discussion in collaborative learning situations.

Simulation

Simulation is used extensively in medical education at all levels, ranging from basic practical skills tuition to scenario-based teaching in a high-fidelity simulator and from simple role play to complex communication skills teaching using simulated patients and actors. Sometimes highly sophisticated, all these teaching methods involve small-group discussion in feedback and to promote reflection. Tutors require high-level specific skills to manage these teaching methods, all of which are grounded in the basic principles required for collaborative and active learning.

Problem-based learning

Problem-based learning (PBL) is a particular form of collaborative learning that has received widespread acceptance in undergraduate medical education. Presentation of clinical material as the stimulus for learning enables students to understand the relevance of underlying scientific knowledge and principles in clinical practice. However, it has implications for curriculum design, staffing and learning resources and demands a different approach to timetabling, workload and assessment.

Generally, PBL is introduced in the context of a defined core curriculum with integration of basic and clinical sciences, often being used to deliver core material in non-clinical parts of the curriculum. Paper-based PBL scenarios form the basis of the core curriculum and ensure that all students are exposed to the same problems. Recently, modified PBL techniques have been introduced into clinical education, with 'real' patients being used as the stimulus for learning. Despite the essential ad hoc nature of learning clinical medicine, a 'key cases' approach can enable PBL to be used to deliver the core clinical curriculum.

In PBL, students use 'triggers' from the problem case scenario to define their own learning objectives. Subsequently, they do an independent, self-directed study before returning to the group to discuss and refine their acquired knowledge. Thus, PBL is not about problem-solving per se, but rather it uses appropriate problems to increase knowledge and understanding. The process is clearly defined, and the several variations that exist all follow a similar series of steps (Box 3.4).

> Box 3.4 **PBL tutorial process**
>
> *Step 1* – Identify and clarify unfamiliar terms presented in the scenario; scribe lists those that remain unexplained after discussion.
>
> *Step 2* – Define the problem or problems to be discussed; students may have different views on the issues, but all should be considered; scribe records a list of agreed problems.
>
> *Step 3* – Discuss the problem(s) at 'brainstorming' sessions, suggesting possible explanations on the basis of prior knowledge; students draw on each other's knowledge and identify areas of incomplete knowledge; scribe records all discussion.
>
> *Step 4* – Review steps 2 and 3 and arrange explanations into tentative solutions; scribe organises the explanations and restructures if necessary.
>
> *Step 5* – Formulate learning objectives; group reaches consensus on the learning objectives; tutor ensures learning objectives are focused, achievable, comprehensive and appropriate.
>
> *Step 6* – Private study (all students gather information related to each learning objective).
>
> *Step 7* – Group shares results of private study (students identify their learning resources and share their results); tutor checks learning and may assess the group.

The PBL tutorial

A typical PBL tutorial consists of a group of students (usually 8 to 10) and a tutor, who facilitates the session. The length of time (number of sessions) that a group stays together with each other and with individual tutors varies between institutions. A group needs to be together long enough to allow good group dynamics to develop but may need to be changed occasionally if personality clashes or other dysfunctional behaviour emerges.

Students elect a chair for each PBL scenario and a 'scribe' to record the discussion. The roles are rotated for each scenario (Figure 3.3). Suitable flip charts or a whiteboard should be used to record the proceedings. At the start of the session, depending on the trigger material, either the student chair reads out the scenario or all students study the material. If the trigger is a real patient in a ward, clinic or surgery, then a student may be asked to take a clinical history or identify an abnormal physical sign before the group moves to a tutorial room. For each module, students may be given a handbook containing the problem scenarios, and suggested learning resources or learning materials may be handed out at appropriate times as the tutorials progress (Box 3.5).

The role of the tutor is to facilitate the proceedings (helping the chair to maintain group dynamics and moving the group through the task) and to ensure that the group achieves appropriate leaning objectives in line with those set by the curriculum design team. The tutor may need to table a more active role in step 7 of the process to ensure that all the students have done the appropriate work and to help the chair to suggest a suitable format for group members to use to present the results of their private study. The tutor should

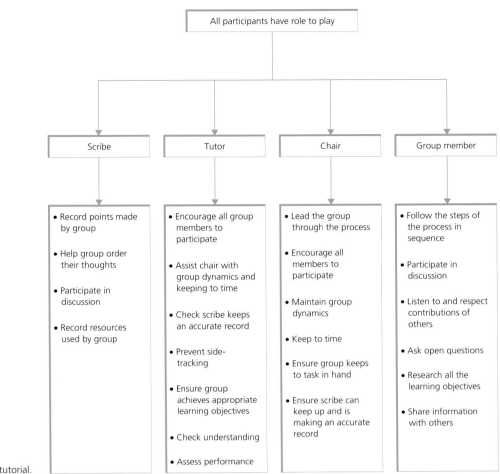

Figure 3.3 Roles of participants in a PBL tutorial.

Box 3.5 **Examples of trigger material for PBL scenarios**

- Paper-based clinical scenarios
- Experimental or clinical laboratory data
- Photographs
- Video clips
- Newspaper articles
- All or part of an article from a scientific journal
- A real or simulated patient
- A family tree showing an inherited disorder

encourage students to check their understanding of the material. He or she can do this by encouraging the students to ask open questions and ask each other to explain topics in their own words or by the use of drawings and diagrams.

Case-based learning

Case-based learning (CBL) is an adaptation of the PBL process and is used more generally in clinical medical education to provide knowledge in context and to offer opportunities for the development of clinical reasoning and judgement. Written case studies,

either prepared by the tutor or brought by group members, present background data and students are required to work together to identify the clinical problems, prepare differential diagnoses and suggest potential investigations and treatment. Students set their own learning objectives and identify the learning resources required to confirm or refute their diagnostic possibilities. The CBL format is flexible and may involve the incorporation of role play or the acquisition of data by gaining further clinical experience to solve the clinical problems.

Peer teaching and community of learners

Peer teaching is widely used in undergraduate medical education, usually in a format whereby one or more senior students are involved in teaching more junior colleagues in either classroom or clinical situations. It facilitates the basic learning of the novice group while promoting learning in the seniors, not only about the topics under consideration but also in relationship to the teaching methods they must themselves employ.

The community of learners methodology is a variation on peer teaching involving guided learning, objective-setting, self-direction and exploration and knowledge exchange to enable problem-solving (Box 3.6).

Box 3.6 **The community of learners method for collaborative learning**

Guided learning (tutor-led)	One or more lectures or tutorials
	Describe the aims of the exercise or course
	Introduce the topic
	Provide the basic knowledge base
	Divide the large group into smaller research groups
	Each research group investigates a different topic
Self-direction and exploration (student-led)	Students work individually using a range of learning resources
	Students communicate regularly within their research group either in meetings or electronically
	Tutor provides expert assistance and progress monitoring for each group
	Groups communicate with other groups to identify their progress
Guided learning (tutor-led)	Intermittent large group sessions to present further information
Knowledge exchange and problem-solving sessions (tutor-led)	Research groups split up and re-form into mixed small groups
	Each mixed group solves a problem that requires knowledge only possessed by the separate research groups

The community of learners method is complex to organise and requires excellent cooperation between student groups, individuals and the tutor. If well-executed it provides students with the opportunities to acquire all the generic skills and attitudes offered by collaborative learning methodologies.

Conclusion

Collaborative learning techniques offer an effective way of delivering medical education with several advantages over traditional didactic teaching methods. All the methods described are based on principles of adult learning theory, including motivating the students, encouraging them to set their own learning goals and giving them a role in decisions that affect their own learning. They can be used within a curriculum either as a sole teaching method or, more usually, in combination with other teaching formats to generate a more stimulating and challenging educational environment, and the beneficial effects from the generic attributes acquired through collaborative and active learning should not be underestimated.

Further reading

Evans D, Brown J. *Working in a group*. In Evans D, Brown J, eds. *How to Succeed at Medical School*. Oxford, UK: BMJ Publishing/Wiley Blackwell, 2009; pp. 71–87.

Hativa N. Teaching methods for active learning. In Hativa N, ed. *Teaching for Effective Learning in Higher Education*. Dordrecht, NL: Kluwer Academic Publishers, 2001; pp. 111–129.

Ramsden P. Teaching strategies for effective learning. In Ramsden P, ed. *Learning to Teach in Higher Education*. London, UK: Routledge, 1992; pp. 150–180.

Srinivasan M, Wilkes M, Stevenson F, Nguyen T, Slavin S. Comparing problem-based learning with case-based learning: effects of a major curricular shift at two institutions. *Academic Medicine* 2007;82:74–82.

CHAPTER 4

Evaluation

Jillian Morrison

University of Glasgow, Glasgow, UK

OVERVIEW

- Evaluation should be a positive process that enables strategic development of a curriculum
- The goals of an evaluation should be clearly articulated and linked to the outcomes of teaching
- More than one source and type of information should be obtained and the results should be fed back to participants with details of the resulting action
- Learners need to be involved in developing an evaluation, to feel that their time is respected and to know that their opinions are valued and acted on
- Evaluators must act on the result of an evaluation to correct deficiencies, improve methods and update content and repeat the process

Evaluation

Evaluation is an essential part of developing any educational experience and can enable educators to find out if the learning events they provide are effective and if not, how they can be improved. The focus of evaluation is on quality improvement and it is necessary to ensure ongoing relevance, coherence, balance and progression within a curriculum. Medical schools and other learning organisations engage in evaluation as part of their own institution's quality assurance processes and also to comply with national processes, for example, Quality Assurance of Basic Medical Education conducted by the General Medical Council (GMC) in the United Kingdom. Evaluation provides evidence about how well students' learning objectives are being achieved and whether teaching standards are being maintained. Crucially, it also ensures that the curriculum evolves to continue to meet the changing needs of students, institutions and society. It should be viewed as a positive process that contributes to the academic development of an institution and its members (Box 4.1).

Box 4.1 **Purposes of evaluation**

- To ensure that teaching is effective in helping students meet their learning outcomes
- To identify areas where teaching can be improved
- To inform the allocation of faculty resources
- To provide feedback and encouragement for teachers
- To support applications for promotion by teachers
- To identify and articulate what is valued by medical schools
- To facilitate development of the curriculum to meet society's needs

Planning an evaluation

Evaluation should ideally be planned at the start of developing a learning experience, not added as an afterthought. The questions asked at the stage of developing an evaluation are similar to those that should be asked when developing a research project (Box 4.2). However, although evaluation and research are similar activities, there are some important differences. Research is usually aimed at producing generalisable results that can be published in peer-reviewed literature and it requires ethical approval. Evaluation is usually carried out for local use and does not usually require ethics approval, although it should be carefully reviewed by curriculum committees to ensure that it is carried out ethically and there are no unintended adverse consequences. Finally, evaluation is a continuous process or cycle of quality improvement, whereas

Box 4.2 **Questions to ask when planning an evaluation**

- What are the goals of the evaluation?
- Who are the stakeholders in the evaluation?
- What should be evaluated and what information should be collected?
- What methods will be used to collect the information?
- From whom will the information be collected?
- Who will collect and analyse the information?
- How will the information be fed back to the stakeholders?
- What decisions can be made as a result of the evaluation?
- When will the evaluation be repeated?

ABC of Learning and Teaching in Medicine, 2nd edition.
Edited by Peter Cantillon and Diana Wood. © 2010 Blackwell Publishing Ltd.

LIBRARY
EDUCATION CENTRE
PRINCESS ROYAL HOSPITAL

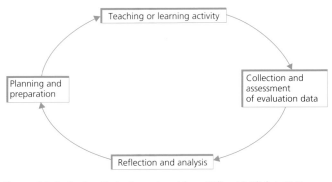

Figure 4.1 Evaluation Cycle. Reproduced from Wilkes M, Bligh J. *BMJ* 1999;318:1269–1272, with permission from BMJ Publishing Group Ltd.

research may be complete if the answer to the research question is answered satisfactorily (Figure 4.1).

What are the goals of the evaluation?

When an educational need has been identified, the first stage of planning is to define the learning outcomes for the curriculum that will address that learning need. The goals of the evaluation should be linked to the learning outcomes and clearly articulated. For example, if the learning outcome of an educational event is that students should be competent in a particular clinical skill, the goal of the evaluation might be to determine if the event enabled the students to achieve that skill effectively. Clarifying the goals of the evaluation makes it much easier to specify the evidence needed to determine success or failure of the teaching. An evaluation protocol should then be prepared so that individual responsibilities are clearly outlined.

Who are the stakeholders in the evaluation?

The stakeholders are determined by the purpose of the evaluation. They usually include students and may also include teachers, current and future patients and institutions. Society may also have an interest, for example, is the tax payer receiving value for money from medical education?

What should be evaluated and what information should be collected?

The resources devoted to evaluation should reflect its importance, but excessive data collection should be avoided. A good system should be easy to administer and should use some information that is readily available.

Evaluation may cover the educational process and/or the outcome of any aspect of education but often focuses on the delivery and content of teaching. Questions about delivery may relate to organisation, for example, administrative arrangements, physical environment, teaching methods and aptitude of the teacher(s) involved. The content of teaching may be evaluated for its level

Self-evaluation	Peer evaluation
• Academic staff increasingly evaluate their own teaching practice • Self-evaluation is useful if the objective is to provide motivation to change behaviour • To help define what they are doing, teachers may find it useful to use videotapes made during teaching, logbooks and personal portfolios	• Direct observation of teachers by their peers can provide an informed, valuable and diagnostic evaluation • Mutual classroom exchange visits between trusted colleagues can be valuable to both the teacher and the observer

Figure 4.2 Participation by teachers in evaluation.

(neither too easy nor too difficult), its relevance to curriculum objectives and how it integrates with previous learning.

In recent times, evaluation has come to play an increasing role in appraising teachers (Figure 4.2).

Kirkpatrick described four levels on which to focus outcome evaluation (Box 4.3); these have been adapted for use in health education evaluation by Barr and colleagues (Barr *et al.* 2000). In practice, outcome measures usually show the impact of the curriculum on the knowledge and skills of students. Some indication of these attributes may be obtained by specific methods of enquiry – for example, by analysing data from student assessments. Unfortunately, evaluation less commonly addresses the top levels of the hierarchy.

> **Box 4.3 Kirkpatrick's four levels on which to focus evaluation**
>
> • Level 1 – Learner's reactions
> • Level 2a – Modification of attitudes and perceptions
> • Level 2b – Acquisition of knowledge and skills
> • Level 3 – Change in behaviour
> • Level 4a – Change in organisational practice
> • Level 4b – Benefits to patients or clients
>
> Adapted by Barr *et al.* 2000. Reproduced by permission of CAIPE.

What methods will be used to collect the information?

An ideal evaluation method would be reliable, valid, acceptable and inexpensive. However, establishing the reliability and validity of instruments and methods of evaluation can take many years and be costly. Testing and retesting of instruments to establish their psychometric properties without any additional benefit for students and teachers is unlikely to be popular with them. Evaluators should

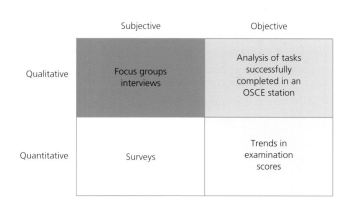

	Subjective	Objective
Qualitative	Focus groups interviews	Analysis of tasks successfully completed in an OSCE station
Quantitative	Surveys	Trends in examination scores

Figure 4.3 Examples of methods of evaluation.

look for 'off-the-shelf' instruments that can be used to evaluate curricula reliably. Apart from the characteristics of an ideal method mentioned above, the process of evaluation itself may produce a positive educational impact if it emphasises those elements that are considered valuable and important by institutions.

Methods used may involve subjective and objective measures and qualitative and quantitative approaches. Quantitative approaches help to answer 'how much' questions and qualitative approaches help to answer 'why' questions. More than one source and method of information should be sought, so that findings can be triangulated (Figure 4.3).

Interviews – Individual interviews with students are useful if the information is sensitive – for example, when a teacher has received poor ratings from students and the reasons are unclear. A group interview (or focus group) can provide detailed views from students or teachers. A teaching session can end with reflection by the group on process issues.

Surveys – Questionnaires are useful for obtaining information from large numbers of students or teachers about the teaching process. Electronic methods for administering questionnaires may improve response rates and can make data input and analysis much easier. The quality of the information, however, is only as good as the questions asked, and while the rating for a learning experience may be available from a simple questionnaire survey, the reasons for a good or a poor rating may not be clear. In other words, a questionnaire might highlight strengths and weaknesses but not answer the 'why' questions.

Information from student assessment – Data from assessment are useful for finding out if students have achieved the learning outcomes of a curriculum. A downward trend in examination results over several cohorts of students may indicate a deficiency in the curriculum. Caution is needed, however, when interpreting this source of information, as students' examination performance depends on their application, ability and motivation as well as on the teaching.

From whom will the information be collected?

To reduce possible bias in evaluation, the views of more than one group of people should be collected. Any of the stakeholders may provide information but in practice most is obtained from students. There are several important issues that need to be considered when designing an evaluation that collects information from students.

Competence – Students can be a reliable and valid source of information. They are uniquely aware of what they are being taught and they observe teaching daily. Daily contact, however, does not mean that they are skilled in evaluation and they need to be briefed about how to give constructive feedback to teachers and curriculum developers. Evaluation by students should also be limited to areas in which they are competent to judge. The relevance of a topic may not be fully apparent to students until they qualify.

Ownership – Students who are not committed to an evaluation may provide poor information. They need to feel ownership of an evaluation by participating in its development, understanding the importance of obtaining the information and what type of information is required, and knowing how it will be used. Usually, the results of an evaluation will affect only subsequent cohorts of students, so current students must be convinced of the value of providing information.

Sampling – Students' time should be respected. If they are asked to fill out endless forms they will perceive their time being wasted and the reliability of the information they provide will deteriorate. One solution is to use different sampling strategies for evaluating different elements of the curriculum. If reliable information can be obtained from 100 students, why collect data from 300?

Anonymity or not – Anonymity is commonly advocated as a guard against bias when information is collected from students. However, asking students to sign evaluation forms can help to create a climate of responsible peer review. If students are identifiable from the information they provide, this must not affect their progress in any way. Information should be collected centrally and students' names removed so that they cannot be identified by teachers they have criticised.

Who will collect and analyse the information?

It is good practice to have the evaluation carried out by colleagues who are not involved in the development and delivery of the curriculum so that the results are free from bias. If this is not possible due to resource constraints, electronic collection and automatic analysis can help. The final results should be discussed with students and others providing the information to ensure that they are valid and accurately reflect their views.

How will information be fed back to the stakeholders?

Students and other stakeholders who provide information need to know that their opinions are respected, so they should be informed of the results of the evaluation as closely as possible to the time of collecting the information. Even if the students have moved on to the next stage in their education, they should still be told about the action that will be taken as a result of the evaluation as this will encourage them to be involved again in the future.

What decisions can be made as a result of the evaluation?

Curriculum developers need to be committed to changing aspects of their course provision that do not meet stakeholders' needs. Collecting information that persistently highlights the same deficiency at every evaluation cycle with no attempt to improve it suggests that developers are going through the motions of evaluation. However, asking for feedback about something that cannot be changed is wasting stakeholder's time. It is extremely useful to have thought about what changes can be made as a result of evaluation before designing the content of an evaluation so that expectations are not raised. For example, asking students to give their preferred day of the week for a teaching session when there is no possibility of changing the timetable is wasting everyone's time.

When will the evaluation be repeated?

The time to repeat the collection of evaluation information depends on how long it will take to analyse and reflect on the information obtained and to implement any required changes. A process for reviewing evaluation and agreeing on course changes needs to be built into the staff timetable so that it happens automatically. For example, course information that is collected on an annual basis can be reviewed during the summer term and changes developed and implemented in time for the new academic session in medical schools, but staff need to be aware that this is a responsibility during the summer.

Completing the evaluation cycle

The main purpose of evaluation is to inform curriculum development. No curriculum is perfect in design and delivery. If the results of an evaluation suggest that no further development is required, doubt must be cast on the process of evaluation. This does not mean that curriculums should be in a constant state of change, but that the evaluation information is acted on and that the curriculum continues to improve. Then the process starts all over again (Box 4.4).

Box 4.4 **Real example**

In response to GMC recommendations, a new 10-week 'Preparation-for-Practice' course is introduced for final year medical students after their final examinations. The course is designed to improve the confidence of students before starting their first clinical post. Two weeks at the start and two weeks at the end are lectures and workshops on campus and in the middle six weeks students are placed in the hospitals where they will undertake their first clinical post.

Goals of the evaluation – to determine what has worked well in the course and what has not worked so well and whether the students'

---

confidence has improved, so that the course can be adapted if necessary for next year.

Stakeholders – the students undertaking the evaluation, faculty staff who have designed the course and deliver the lectures and workshops and the junior and senior doctors and other hospital staff who support the students on placement.

What should be evaluated – the process of both the campus-based and hospital-based parts of the course and the outcome regarding the confidence of the students.

Methods and subjects – a standard course evaluation form used for evaluation of individual sessions and attachments by students; faculty staff asked to provide comments about their sessions; focus groups carried out with a sample of students immediately after the block and at the end of the first clinical post; interviews conducted with a sample of hospital staff; and an off-the-shelf questionnaire to assess confidence applied to students at the start and end of the course.

Collection and analysis – an evaluation team is formed and opportunistic and planned evaluation sessions are scheduled. A student who is undertaking a Student-Selected Component in Medical Education Evaluation and a Clinical Teaching Fellow based in one of the participating hospitals join the evaluation team and will use the experience as a basis for project dissertations. An external expert is approached for help with analysis of the before- and after-evaluation confidence questionnaires.

Feeding back results – it is agreed that a brief summary report including proposed changes as a result of the evaluation will be produced and distributed to participants. The results will also be discussed at faculty and staff–student meetings.

Decisions – as this is the first time that the new course has been introduced, it is agreed that the course can be completely changed if it does not improve students' confidence and no arrangements are made for the following year until the evaluation information is available.

Repeating the evaluation – it is agreed that the evaluation will be repeated at the end of the following academic session and there will be particular interest in the aspects of the course that are changed in response to the previous year's evaluation.

Further reading

Goldie J. AMEE Education Guide no. 29: evaluating educational programmes. *Medical Teacher* 2006;28:210–224.

Robson C. *Small Scale Evaluation*. London: Sage, 2000.

Snell L, Tallett S, Haist S, Hays R, Norcini J, Prince K *et al*. A review of the evaluation of clinical teaching: new perspectives and challenges. *Medical Education* 2000;34:862–870.

Wilkes M, Bligh J. Evaluating educational interventions. *BMJ* 1999;318: 1269–1272.

Reference

Barr H, Freeth D, Hammick M, Koppel I, Reeves S. *Evaluations of Interprofessional Education: A United Kingdom Review of Health and Social Care*. London: CAIPE/BERA, 2000.

CHAPTER 5

Teaching Large Groups

Peter Cantillon

National University of Ireland, Galway, Ireland

'College is a place where a professor's lecture notes go straight to the students' lecture notes, without passing through the brains of either'

– Mark Twain

OVERVIEW

- Lecturing represents a teaching approach in which the teacher does most, if not all, of the talking irrespective of the group size
- Lectures are often regarded as being an efficient teaching method, yet students retain only 5–10% of what they hear in a traditional lecture
- Lectures are best used for stimulating interest in a subject, providing a framework to support students' understanding and directing further learning
- An effective lecturer is one who aims to stimulate thinking and facilitate learning rather than 'transmit' knowledge
- Teachers need to learn how to use active learning techniques in the design and delivery of their lectures so that they may promote more effective learning

Bad press

Lectures have had a bad press. They are regarded as a 'traditional' form of teaching and are often viewed as being out of step with the newer enquiry-based learning approaches. Where lectures used to be the cornerstone of a curriculum, they are increasingly regarded as pedagogical anachronisms from another age. Lectures were thought to be efficient; they made it possible for relatively few staff to 'teach' large groups of students and to 'cover' large blocks of curriculum. They were thought to be effective based on an assumption that attendance at lectures guaranteed learning. However, traditional lectures encourage learner passivity and there is good evidence to show that learners retain very little (5~10%) of what they hear in lectures.

The place of lectures in a modern medical curriculum

Large-group teaching (or lecturing) is about an approach to teaching rather than the actual numbers of students in an audience. It is

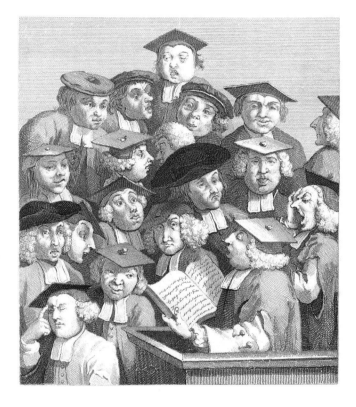

quite possible to 'lecture' 10 students in a tutorial group. Lecturing represents a form of teaching in which the teacher controls the content and does most (if not all) of the talking. However, despite their bad press, lectures do have important roles in an educational programme. For example, lecturers represent an excellent means of

- introducing a new subject;
- demonstrating how knowledge is structured and prioritised in a particular domain;
- stimulating curiosity;
- directing further study;
- linking research and practice.

ABC of Learning and Teaching in Medicine, 2nd edition.
Edited by Peter Cantillon and Diana Wood. © 2010 Blackwell Publishing Ltd.

If lectures are to have an important place in a curriculum, the challenge for teachers is to ensure that students learn more and derive better value from attending lectures. It has been well shown that learner passivity is no more likely in large-group teaching than in small group or bedside teaching if lecturers employ techniques that encourage active learning (see Box 5.1) amongst their students. What is required is a change of attitude. Lecturing should no longer be about performance or transmitting knowledge; rather, an effective lecturer is one who aims to stimulate thinking and facilitate student learning. The remainder of this chapter will discuss how preparing, delivering and evaluating lectures can all be enhanced through active learning.

Box 5.1 **Active learning**

Active learning is not, as its name suggests, about keeping students busy. Active learning is an approach to teaching in which the teacher recognises that it is the learner who does the learning and therefore makes every effort to facilitate that process. In other words, teaching is about facilitating the process of learning rather than transmitting information. Typically, in an active learning context, the learner is encouraged to become more aware of what he/she knows and to elaborate his/her knowledge through thinking, dialogue and engagement with the subject matter. The teacher's role is to facilitate the learner in constructing new understandings and better knowledge. This is often stated as a change of teaching roles from the 'sage on the stage' to the 'guide on the side'.

Planning for active learning in lectures

One of the first steps, therefore, in planning a lecture is to gain access to the student study guides or curricular documents to get some idea about what students already know or have experienced. It is also important to talk to other teachers who teach within the same year and to speak to students about what they have covered and where the gaps lie.

When planning lecture content, the most important thing is to identify the critical concepts and principles that underpin everything else. These are usually the concepts and principles that are essential for solving problems in the domain. It is also important to identify the so-called 'difficult concepts' that students find hard to understand and learn. Talking to other teachers, speaking to past students and looking at previous student assessment performance can reveal the concepts and principles that students find difficult to master. Difficult concepts require special attention in lectures with the incorporation of powerful analogies, examples and the provision of opportunities for students to demonstrate their understanding.

Once a lecture has been written, it is important to review its content and to make a conscious effort to reduce it to an essential core. 'Less is more' is a good axiom when planning lectures. Students are frequently overwhelmed by content in lectures. There is little time to process new information before the next slide is shown and much content is missed because students cannot listen and write at the same time. Teachers need to trust that learners will add to the minimal core knowledge they acquire in lectures through further study and learning in other settings. The important task for lecturers, therefore, is to identify the subject's core knowledge and concepts and to ensure that learners have a good understanding by the end of the lecture.

Students like handouts. Most lecturers make their PowerPoint slides available to students, but slides often represent bullet point knowledge and are not that effective as revision tools or stimulators of student thinking. Good handouts, on the other hand, can fulfil several functions. They can highlight key points, they illustrate relationships, they can provide materials for student exercises during class and they can direct further learning through questions, challenges and reading lists (see Box 5.2 on designing handouts).

Box 5.2 **Designing handouts**

Handouts should provide scaffolding on which the students can build their understanding of a topic. Thus if a handout provides all of the information contained in a lecture, students are unlikely to pay too much attention to what the lecturer says and may spend their time doing a crossword or doodling at the side of a page. Handouts should provide a summary of the major themes while avoiding an exhaustive explanation of each. Thus, the best handouts are usually a brief summary of what the lecture contains with partially completed diagrams, questions for further study and recommendations for further reading. Handouts should encourage students to spend more time listening and less time writing notes; in other words, handouts should be about encouraging students to listen and think rather than write and miss essential explanations of difficult concepts.

Active learning in lectures

Without attention, there is no learning. Teachers need to design activities to grab students' attention early in lectures. There are some well-known techniques:

- Ask the students to solve a 'concrete' problem at the start of a lecture. By applying their common sense to the problem they will come to understand what they know about the subject and also what they need to know and this makes them more likely to pay attention.
- Show the students a video or case presentation that illustrates or exemplifies key parts of the lecture content. This will act as a means of letting the students know what they are going to learn and helps them focus their thinking.
- Give the students a small test or quiz so that they can assess their knowledge at the start of lecture. The same quiz can be delivered again at the end of the lecture to demonstrate both to them and to the lecturer what has been learnt.

Signposting

As stated above, students are often overwhelmed by content in lectures. Learners cannot see the gestalt or big picture of a subject in the same way as a teacher can. 'Signposting' is a technique in which teachers tell students at the start what they are going to be able to do by the end of the lecture (the learning objectives) and provide a lecture outline that indicates the structure of the lecture at regular intervals during the lecture.

Students often miss vital bits of lectures because of temporary inattention, for example, when they are writing notes. Summaries at regular intervals in lectures provide a means for learners to catch up. Other related approaches include allowing students 3–5 minute breaks in lectures to make notes or giving them exercises in class that are designed to reinforce what they have just heard and learnt.

Active learning techniques

In recognition of the fact that students' attention tends to wane, teachers should attempt to deliver lectures in chunks or phases, punctuated with exercises, challenges and questions to stimulate knowledge processing and elaboration. It is good, therefore, to plan a lecture in 10- or 15-minute chunks with 5-minute breaks for note taking and exercises. The following represent some of the many exercises and techniques that can be used to stimulate active learning in large-group settings:

- The in-class quiz is a brief test (e.g. an MCQ) delivered and corrected during class time. In-class quizzes can be used for many purposes including getting attention at the start of a lecture and assessing how well students have grasped a subject at the end of the lecture.
- Audience response systems (or 'clickers') represent an increasingly common active learning tool used in large-class settings. Clickers are hand-held devices that allow students to indicate their responses to surveys of class opinion, for example, in response to challenging questions posed by the teacher. The results appear on the screen as a bar chart or graph demonstrating the distribution of student responses. Audience response systems can be excellent for stimulating thought and encouraging debate among students about alternative responses to complex topics. They can also provide a means of looking at how students perform during in-class quizzes.
- Brainstorm is an excellent technique for encouraging students to think about a topic before the teacher provides his/her perspective. Brainstorm is an exercise in which the lecturer asks the students to generate answers or suggestions to a problem or topic (see Figure 5.1). The lecturer writes the students' responses without comment onto a white board, flipchart or blackboard. Brainstorming usually ends with the lecturer attempting to organise and collate the ideas and suggestions offered by students.
- Buzz groups represent an exercise in which a lecturer asks the class to work in groups of two to four to solve problems or answer challenging questions. They are known as 'buzz' groups because of the amount of noise that they generate in a lecture. It is usual to allow buzz groups to work on a problem for several minutes and then to call the lecture to order. A good way to ensure that the buzz groups have been working meaningfully is for the teacher

to indicate that one or two buzz groups will be asked to report back to the whole group on what they have discussed and agreed on in their group.

- Questioning is a commonly used technique in which either the teacher asks questions of the class or the teacher encourages the class to ask questions. An important technique when asking questions is to use the so-called 'ten-second rule'. Students feel intimidated about speaking up in large-group settings; thus it is useful to count to 10 before prompting the audience for a response to a question or selecting a 'volunteer'. A good technique for dealing with student reticence when prompted to ask questions of the teacher is to instruct students to try out their questions on each other in buzz groups or pairs before selecting their best question for the lecturer.
- Bringing patients to a lecture can be very stimulating for students. Presenting a case and then engaging the patient in a demonstration of aspects of history taking or asking the patient to interact with students about their experiences of a particular disease can be hugely beneficial.
- Class debates can be used for controversial topics so that students can begin to understand the issues from different perspectives. Students are asked to elect speakers for and against a 'motion'. The teacher keeps time and the class adjudicate with a show of hands. Debates represent an excellent method of engaging students' attention; it is important, however, to allow time at the end to summarise what has been learnt and to deal with any misconceptions or inconsistencies.

Active learning has major implications for the use of time in lectures. A typical 50-minute lecture may require several breaks for exercises, summaries and note taking. Thus, for example, in a 50-minute lecture, teachers might need to anticipate 35 minutes of talk time and 15 minutes for questions, class exercises and note taking (Box 5.3).

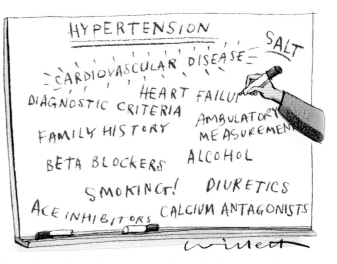

Figure 5.1 Brainstorming is a useful technique for focusing students' attention.

Box 5.3 **Things that lecturers do that undermine learning activity**

1. Excessive content
2. Delivery too quick (students cannot write and listen at the same time)
3. Poor sequencing
4. Failure to clarify objectives from the start
5. Poor visual aids
6. Handouts that contain 100% of the information contained in the lecture, thus ensuring low attendance and attention
7. Key concepts and points not emphasised, creating a sense of an enormous topic
8. Not paying attention to what the learners already know
9. Not checking understanding afterwards
10. Speaking in one flow with no breaks

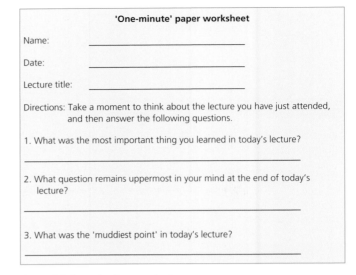

Figure 5.2 Example of a one-minute paper.

Evaluating lectures: an active learning approach

By the end of a lecture the teacher needs to know the answers to a few important questions:

- What have the students learnt?
- Were the lecture and the teaching approach effective?

Let us look at these questions in turn, highlighting a few simple techniques.

What have students learnt?

- The lecturer can ask a few students to show him/her their lecture notes. These can be quite revealing about what students identified as important in the lecture content and can also demonstrate areas of woolly thinking or misconception. A further embellishment is to provide feedback to students who volunteer their notes.
- Students can be asked to complete a 'one-minute paper'. A one-minute paper (see Figure 5.2) is a tool in which you ask students to indicate what was the most important thing they learnt, what questions remain uppermost in their minds at the end of the lecture and what was the muddiest point in the lecture (see example in Figure 5.2). The one-minute paper provides an excellent way of highlighting difficult concepts with which students are struggling, but it also emphasises what from a students' perspective were the most salient messages. Another version of the one-minute paper is to ask students to list the three most important things they learnt during the lecture and to compare them to the three most important things identified by the lecturer.
- Another means of finding out what students have learnt is to carry out a mini-assessment in the last 10 minutes of a lecture. Students are issued with a problem to solve, a diagram to complete or an MCQ that they must complete in 5 minutes. The remaining time can be devoted to presenting solutions, discussing alternatives and fielding questions. Teachers should

also take note of students' achievements on end-of-semester assessments that test the students' mastery of the lecture's learning objectives.

Evaluating the lecturer and teaching effectiveness

- One of the most powerful ways of evaluating a lecture is through peer observation. Peer evaluation represents an evaluation approach in which a colleague observes a lecturer teach and gives feedback according to an agreed rubric or evaluation form. Peer evaluation forms are readily available on the internet and are usually available from centres of learning and teaching within academic institutions. It is important to set time aside after the lecture to receive feedback from the academic peer and to discuss the discrepancies between what was intended and what actually happened.
- The commonest form of evaluation is a student feedback questionnaire. This is usually a quantitative tool designed to assess whether students enjoyed a lecture and understood what was being communicated. The problem with the questionnaires is that students are rather jaded with quantitative surveys. An interesting alternative is to use a short qualitative interview with students after a lecture.

Further reading

Bligh DA. *What's the Use of Lectures?* San Francisco: Jossey-Bass, 2000.

Brown G, Manogue M. AMEE medical education guide no. 22: refreshing lecturing: a guide for lecturers. *Medical Teacher* 2001;23:231–244.

Gibbs G, Habeshaw T. *Preparing to Teach*. Bristol: Technical and Educational Services, 1989.

Newble DI, Cannon R. *A Handbook for Medical Teachers*. 4th ed. Dordrecht, Netherlands: Kluwer Academic, 2001.

CHAPTER 6

Teaching Small Groups

David Jaques

Staff and Educational Development Association, London, UK
Higher Education Academy, London, UK

OVERVIEW

- Group discussion, effectively practised, can help develop a range of skills such as self-expression, listening collaboration and problem-solving, among students
- Attention to group size and membership can play a significant part in the success of group learning
- Groups of different sizes tend to display quite different dynamics
- Self-assessment of their own participation can help students develop awareness of their skills in a group
- Reflection through self-evaluation by tutors can equally help in developing their role
- Tutors may find it helpful to recognise and consciously work with some of a group's typical developmental stages
- Independent group work can help students learn about leadership and teamwork issues
- An agreed set of ground rules can enhance group management
- Regular reviews of the group's progress help in sharing responsibility for its success

- It presents challenges to personal beliefs and assumptions.
- It develops positive and informed attitudes to collaborative work.
- It develops skills in problem-solving, teamwork, evaluating and decision-making.
- It places the teacher in a position to identify the relative strengths and weaknesses of students and thus to give attention to relevant support and change.

Group composition and size

Choices in the size and membership of groups can be important factors in successful discussion.

As a general rule, a heterogeneous mix provides the best combination for interaction and achievement of task. Such qualities as age, sex, culture and personality may be taken into account, though one can never be sure what specific mixture will lead to effective participation. Individual members will contribute differently according to who they are grouped with (and what the sitting arrangements are), sometimes producing what is known as an 'assembly effect' – a subconscious convergence of needs and behaviours, which is often impossible to predict. Indeed the leader may be part of it, for example, when a group of dependent participants is led by an authoritative or charismatic person.

Whether from the point of view of learning or problem-solving or decision-making, the mixing of quicker or more perceptive students with their slower counterparts can enable a teaching/learning process between the students to take place (given suitable ground rules and tasks). Often the most powerful influences are the personal likes and dislikes of fellow members. People tend to agree with individuals they like and disagree with those they dislike even though both may express the same opinion. There is clearly some place for process observations from the tutor here.

Groups may be led by either a tutor or a student member or, in some cases, with no one designated and the leadership allowed to circulate or be shared.

With project or task teams both the size of the group and its composition will need special attention. Small groups may lack the necessary variety of expertise to achieve a dynamic climate, while larger groups may prove more difficult to hold together and be dominated by one or two members. Who should decide the

Small-group discussion, whether face-to-face, online or a blend of the two, has a critical role to play in medical education. When effectively practised, group discussion can contribute significantly to the quality of learning through a balance of mutual support and/or competitive stimulus. Much of its success depends on the practice and development of skills – presenting, listening, critical thinking, collaboration and problem-solving – as well as shared values, as indicated in Box 6.1.

Box 6.1 **What makes learning in small groups so important?**

- It creates a collective learning context.
- It increases tolerance for complexity, uncertainty and ambiguity.
- It enables exploration of a range/diversity of views.
- It develops the skills of giving and handling feedback.
- It encourages respectful listening for understanding.

ABC of Learning and Teaching in Medicine, 2nd edition.
Edited by Peter Cantillon and Diana Wood. © 2010 Blackwell Publishing Ltd.

membership and how? While self-chosen groups may have their merits they may lead to some kind of conformity of interests and abilities; teams of friends may collude in not challenging each other. A carefully balanced group membership using Belbin's team roles (see Jaques and Salmon 2006, p. 153) can be followed by negotiated changes where individual students make a case for them.

Student-led groups

There are occasions, planned and otherwise, when it is appropriate to establish groups led and organised by students. Sometimes this may be for practical reasons such as maintaining a small-group format by dividing them when student numbers are large, or because of the absence of suitable tutors or rooms, or even as a strategy towards independent group work. On the other hand, it may be for more educational reasons such as independent learning in project groups.

Small groups compared with large groups

The smaller the group, the greater is the likelihood of close relationships, full participation and consonance of aims. In a small group, roles are likely to be shared or rotated. Five to seven members are generally regarded as the optimum for leaderless groups. In the case of tutor-led groups, and for discussion purposes, groups of 15 tend to be the largest sizes for reasonably full participation. By dividing and arranging larger groups into smaller units, however, we can make the tasks of learning and its management both less demanding and less problematical, an example being that of breaking into pairs at times when the discussion is likely to get stuck (Table 6.1).

Because of their natural tendency to differentiate roles, equality is harder to achieve in larger groups, a factor that is as likely to apply to both online and face-to-face situations. Structured activities (q.v.) where larger groups break into smaller ones while still maintaining a sense of the whole group can provide the best features of both. Online, groups do not find it easy to work virtually, so without careful structuring, and the use of active and interactive 'e-tivities'

(Salmon 2002), it is unlikely that discussion will move beyond sharing information, support and encouragement. E-tivities are based largely on participants 'making sense' of material through interaction with their peers and with their e-moderators. Online equalness is usually easier to achieve as no one has to wait a turn, and shy people can blossom. Be careful with humour and irony – it does not work so well until participants are very comfortable, and offence can be taken.

Brookfield and Preskill suggest the following four approaches to inclusivity in groups:

1 *Begin discussion with some form of personal disclosure* such as individual experiences, enthusiasms and fears so that the students feel they know each other. *Group rounds*, where everyone in turn is given 20 seconds or so to say anything they noticed, thought or learnt about the topic (or would like to learn) without interruption and *paired introductions* (interviewing and introducing a partner) are useful devices here.
2 *Encourage ground rules that make it OK for everyone to stumble in conversation*, miss the point and so on without feeling discredited; teachers (tutors) can help by modelling this.
3 *Call time-outs* to allow students to review and connect points that have been made with their experiences.
4 *Introduce periods of women-only discussion*, possibly alternating with men-only periods, and comparing the two.

Management of students in groups

Although working in small groups may seem to be a welcome break for students from the routine of classroom teaching, we have to recognise that some may behave as if this was not the case, and act in ways that compromise the group's effectiveness, for example, by opting out either physically or mentally with a resentful attitude because they strongly prefer to work alone. Others may characteristically dominate, by speaking too much, not listening to others. We must also recognise that some students may dislike working in groups for reasons of rivalry (not wanting others to benefit from their input) or feelings of inadequacy (which may be intellectual or psychological).

Ground rules

While we can address some of the above behaviours through effective 'chairing' of the group, we should recognise that some of the above conflict and withdrawal behaviours may well emanate from the tutor being seen as an authority figure. For these reasons, it may make sense to 'delegate' the tutor's chairing role via some ground rules such as those in Box 6.2.

Ground rules can also be generated by the group through a group exercise, perhaps in pairs, focusing on the students' experiences of what helps and hinders discussion and what the group might do to encourage and avoid them (Brookfield and Preskill 2005; pp. 53–56). The last two rules provided in Box 6.2 are two meta-rules that might be added sensibly.

Table 6.1 How the experience of large groups is likely to differ from that of small groups.

Small groups (3–5)	Larger groups (6–15)
Close relationships	Some close, some distant
Agreement on aims	Variety of aims
Can be too cosy	Can be challenging
Limited range of views	Wider range of views
Roles naturally shared or rotated	Roles emerge
More intimate	More detached
Coherence	Fragmentation occurs
Full participation likely	Leadership or rules needed to hold group together
Equality ⟵⟶	**Differentiation**

Box 6.2 **Ground rules**

- We start and finish on time.
- We come prepared for the discussion.
- The shared aim is to listen and understand each other.
- Everyone has some responsibility for the process and the achievement of group aims: therefore it is up to everyone, not just the tutor, to bring in other members of the group.
- When anyone speaks, they are addressing the whole group and not just the tutor.
- Use the word 'I' to begin the contributions where possible.
- We present reasons for disagreeing.
- We criticise others' arguments but not them as persons.
- We may find it helpful to paraphrase what the previous speaker said.
- We listen in order to understand.
- We respond to others as well as initiate new threads.
- Silence is okay, especially if it allows space for others to contribute or for all to think.
- We look for recurring themes and prevailing issues.
- We ask for clarification if necessary.

- *All group members accept these ground rules.*
- *Anyone can remind the group when these rules are not being sensibly observed.*

A seven-stage model of group development

Many of the classic studies of group development have involved group leaders who took a passive or non-directive role and did not directly intervene in the group process (Johnson and Johnson 1987), and this contrasts with the typical tutor-led group in higher education. They propose the following seven-stage model for learning groups where there is a leader with clear responsibility for the effective functioning of the group:

1. Defining and structuring procedures
At the first meeting, the group will expect the tutor/leader to explain what is expected of them, what the plan and purpose of the meetings is and how the group is going to operate (whether this is fulfilled is of course a matter of choice). Typically with a learning group, the tutor will clarify the task, explain procedures and generally set-up the group in readiness for its work together.

2. Conforming to procedures and getting acquainted
As the group members get used to the procedures and norms of the group, they also become more familiar and relaxed with each other. The group is still dependent on the tutor for direction and the members are happy to conform according to the process norms of the group whether explicitly or implicitly expressed. They do not yet feel a personal commitment to the group's goals or to each other.

3. Recognising mutuality and building trust
The group members begin to recognise their interdependence and to build a sense of cooperation and trust. They internalise the sense that group learning is a collaborative venture and participate actively in discussions. There is a feeling of mutual support and trust.

4. Rebelling and differentiating
This stage represents a pulling back from the previous two as members start to resist the responsibilities they had apparently accepted and become counter-dependent, contravening many of the group-learning procedures. Sometimes, this may mean returning to a more passive, minimal effort role and forgetting the previously held cooperative ethos. Despite its apparent negativity, this stage is important for members in establishing interpersonal boundaries and a sense of autonomy which can lead to a stronger, because self-owned, collaboration. Johnson and Johnson suggest that tutors should regard this rebellion and conflict as natural and 'deal with both in an open and accepting way'. They recommend not tightening control and trying to force conformity: reasoning and negotiating; confronting and problem-solving; mediating conflicts while helping to underpin autonomy and individuality; working towards participants taking ownership of procedures and committing themselves to each other's success. 'Coordinating a learning group is like teaching a child to ride a bicycle', they say. You have to run alongside to prevent the child from falling off, giving the child space and freedom to learn how to balance on his or her own.

5. Committing to and taking ownership for the goals, procedures and other members
The group becomes 'our' group, not the tutor's. The group norms of cooperation become internalised and no longer have to be externally imposed; the members are no longer dependent on the tutor as the driving force, and find support and help from each other. Friendships develop.

6. Functioning maturely and productively
A sense of collaborative identity develops as the group matures into an effective working unit. Group members learn to operate in different ways in order to achieve group goals and can readily alternate attention between task and maintenance concerns. At this stage, they can usually cope with any problems that arise in the group without the help of the tutor who in turn takes on the role of a consultant and resource to the group. Labour is divided according to expertise, members ask for and accept help from each other and leadership is shared among the members.

Johnson and Johnson remark that many discussion groups do not reach this stage either because the tutor does not have the ability to establish cooperative interdependence or group members do not collectively possess the necessary skills to function in this way. Part of the tutor's job is therefore to ensure that group members are acquiring the skills they need to progress to this stage.

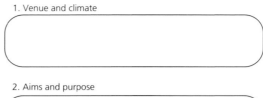
LIBRARY
EDUCATION CENTRE
PRINCESS ROYAL HOSPITAL

Does the tutor.......

Ensure the venue is suitable in
terms of seating, heating, lighting etc.?
Establish a congenial atmosphere in which
students' viewpoints are valued?

1. Venue and climate

Ensure that students understand
the aims of the session(s)? And how
these relate to other parts of their course?
And what they can expect to achieve
from the session(s)?

2. Aims and purpose

Make sure the students know what is
expected of them by way of preparation?
That they understand when it is appropriate
to contribute, to raise a question or to
challenge points made by others?

3. Ground rules

Select tasks appropriate to the aims
of the session? Do the tasks offer the
students a variety of learning experiences
(e.g. the chance to draw on their own
resources and experiences, but also share
with and learn from others)?

4. Planning tasks

Ensure tasks early in the session(s)
enable all to be involved? Make sure
the outcomes from one task lead to
another? Give clear and succinct
instructions? Set and keep to realistic
time allocations for tasks?

5. Structuring and sequencing tasks

Give positive attention to what
students say? Reflect readiness to
listen in verbal responses and in body
language?

6. Listening

Use a variety of questioning strategies
in a sensitive and flexible manner?

7. Questioning

Allow students space to attempt tasks
or think about questions before giving
own explanations? Build students' ideas
into own explanations?

8. Explaining and clarifying

Figure 6.1 Checklist for group-based learning. Adapted from Day K, Grant R, Hounsell D. *Reviewing Your Teaching*. 1998.

Encourage all students in the group
to contribute, to talk to each other (as
well as the tutor)? Avoid dominating
the proceedings? Intervene appropriately
(e.g. to restrain the vociferous, to encourage
the silent, to defuse unhelpful conflict)?

9. Encouraging participation

Act sensitively to students as individuals
(i.e talking into account their backgrounds
and prior knowledge)?

10. Responding to students as individuals

Provide opportunities for the group
to take stock and to review its effectiveness
as a learning group?

11. Monitoring

Make provisions for summing up what has
been achieved? Establish what is necessary
to follow-up the session and consolidate
what has been learned?

12. Closing

Figure 6.1 *continued.*

7. Terminating

Every group has to come to an end and its members have to move on. The more cohesive and mature a group has become, the more sadness will accompany its ending for both members and tutor. The last meeting must deal with this as a recognisable problem and not avoid it as they leave the group to move on to future experiences.

Most groups, if they are developing effectively, which move fairly quickly through the first five stages, devote most time and energy to the mature and productive stage, and then terminate quickly. The skill of the tutor in handing over the 'perceived ownership' of the group's goals and procedures as it moves from the first two stages through the rebellion is of course critical.

Evaluation

Evaluation is of course another form of feedback, but that does not necessarily mean it should emanate only from the students. A little bit of *self-evaluation* for the tutor, using the following checklist might be an instructive source for quiet reflection before and after leading a group discussion (Box 6.3).

More significantly, where evaluation is seen as more of a regular process in which all group members view themselves as contributors and take responsibility for outcomes, there is more chance of change through cooperation. Five minutes set aside at the end of each meeting to review how things went (*what went well, what could we improve, anything else?*) are therefore likely to be of greater benefit to all concerned than any formal, externally applied procedure.

In order to learn from the students about their experience of the group, the form in Figure 6.1 may be suitable and instructive. Processing this, feeding it back to the students and even discussing it with them can provide an added learning bonus for all concerned.

Box 6.3 **Teaching small groups – checklist for tutors**

Read the following list of statements and tick the box which describes your own teaching best.
   Add four statements of your own.

1. I find it easy to learn students' names	❑	❑	❑	❑	❑	I find it hard to learn students' names
2. My sessions start working slowly	❑	❑	❑	❑	❑	My sessions start working quickly
3. I find it easy to get students to contribute	❑	❑	❑	❑	❑	I find it hard to get students to contribute
4. Most students prepare well	❑	❑	❑	❑	❑	Most students prepare poorly
5. I find it easy to keep discussion to the point	❑	❑	❑	❑	❑	I find it hard to keep discussion to the point
6. I find it easy to keep the discussion going	❑	❑	❑	❑	❑	I find it hard to keep the discussion going
7. I speak more than I would like to	❑	❑	❑	❑	❑	I speak less than I would like to
8. I find myself talking to one or two students	❑	❑	❑	❑	❑	I find myself talking to the whole group
9. Sessions lack structure	❑	❑	❑	❑	❑	Sessions are well structured
10. My students seldom express their own views	❑	❑	❑	❑	❑	My students freely express their own views

11. . . . .
12. . . . .
13. . . . .

Further reading

Day K, Grant R, Hounsell D. *Reviewing Your Teaching*. TLA Centre University of Edinburgh, 1998.

Exley K, Dennick R. *Small Group Teaching – Tutorials, Seminars and Beyond*. Abingdon: Routledge, 2004.

Habeshaw S & T, Gibbs G. *53 Interesting Ways to Run Seminars and Tutorials* 1996; TES, 2000. Now on Amazon.co.uk

Tiberius R. *Small Group Teaching – a Trouble-shooting Guide*. London: Kogan Page, 1999.

References

Brookfield S, Preskill S. *Discussion as a Way of Teaching*. San Francisco: Jossey Bass, 2005.

Day K, Grant R, Hounsell D. *Reviewing your Teaching*. Edinburgh: TLA Centre, University of Edinburgh, 1998.

Jaques D, Salmon G. *Learning in Groups – a Handbook for Face-to-face and Online Environments*, Routledge, 2006.

Johnson D, Johnson F. *Joining Together: Group Theory and Group Skills*. Englewood Cliffs: Prentice Hall, 1987.

Salmon G. *E-tivities: The Key to Active Online Learning*. London: Routledge Falmer, 2002.

CHAPTER 7

Feedback in Medical Education: Skills for Improving Learner Performance

Joan Sargeant and Karen Mann

Dalhousie University, Halifax, Nova Scotia, Canada

OVERVIEW

- Providing feedback can be challenging, but receiving and using feedback can be equally challenging
- Feedback is intended to be constructive and guide performance and achievement, not to criticise or judge
- Creating a culture of improvement in learning and workplace settings, where feedback on performance becomes the norm, supports providing constructive feedback
- For feedback providers, the goals are twofold:
  - to increase our own comfort and skill in providing constructive feedback and
  - for the learners, the feedback receivers, to increase their comfort and skill in seeking, receiving and using feedback

---

Introduction

Providing feedback is challenging for teachers and supervisors. Giving effective, constructive feedback is tough, and we, as educators and supervisors working with learners in clinical settings, generally receive little preparation for it. Yet, research shows that providing specific, relevant and timely feedback in a constructive manner can markedly improve learning and performance. It can make a big difference. This chapter sets out to accomplish four goals:

1 Describe the challenges in giving and receiving feedback.
2 Discuss the rationale for providing regular, specific, constructive feedback.
3 Review a helpful definition of feedback.
4 Provide tips for sharing effective feedback to improve learner performance and achievement.

Challenges in feedback: the gap between giving and receiving

*Feedback involves both the giving and receiving, by teachers and learners, and there can be **gulfs** between these.*
— Hattie and Timperley, (2007)

ABC of Learning and Teaching in Medicine, 2nd edition.
Edited by Peter Cantillon and Diana Wood. © 2010 Blackwell Publishing Ltd.

Why does this gap happen?

To answer this question, we need to explore the perspectives of the feedback providers, teachers and supervisors, and the receivers, students and registrars.

> The purpose of feedback is to improve performance and achievement, not to criticise or judge.

Providing feedback

Clinical faculty and supervisors are often unaware of the positive influence which feedback can have upon learning and performance, failing to see that feedback is essential to learner improvement. Moreover, they may perceive constructive or corrective feedback as 'negative' feedback. This can lead to viewing feedback as a negative experience which causes discomfort, rather than a positive one which helps learners to improve. Some are concerned that providing constructive feedback may negatively influence their relationships with learners or learner's self-esteem. Others believe that they lack the skills or resources to deal effectively with learners receiving negative feedback and needing assistance.

Practically speaking, busy clinical wards and offices combined with demanding professional workloads can pose barriers to providing learner feedback. Even with the best of intentions, it often seems difficult to find a quiet time and space to provide feedback to a learner.

For these reasons, we tend to provide constructive feedback rarely. Instead, we may not provide any feedback or provide generalities like 'you're doing fine' or 'no need to worry' which give the learner little information for improvement.

Receiving feedback

Students and residents/registrars report rarely receiving feedback, and when they do, their impression is that it is frequently too late or incomplete to be helpful. Yet, students and registrars also report not recognising feedback when it is provided; feedback is not always obvious.

Receiving feedback can also be problematic. Even the best formulated feedback can appear to fall on deaf ears, or even be rejected outright. Why is this so? Learners have to constantly balance the benefits of receiving feedback with its costs. The benefits include receiving information that will help them perform better and find better ways to reach their goals. The costs may include more work for the learner or the fear of losing face with peers or supervisors. Moreover, learners (and teachers) often go to great lengths to confirm their self-perceptions. They may be more likely therefore to attend to feedback that is congruent with their self-view, and they may reject or ignore accounts of their behaviour that differ from their own.

Feedback can also be given and received at different levels, ranging from comments about the learner's performance of a specific task to perceived criticisms of the self. Feedback which tells learners about their task performance and how they can improve has been shown to have the greatest effect on achievement. Feedback about the self is less useful in improving performance.

Receiving feedback, especially negative feedback, can elicit an emotional response that interferes with accepting the feedback. This is especially so when feedback is perceived as a judgement about 'self', rather than information about how to improve a task.

Other explanations for learners not accepting and using feedback include the following:

- Feedback that is not related to learners' goals or to where they are in relation to those goals
- Feedback that is vague and offers no cues for how to improve
- Feedback that is not perceived as credible; for example, learners may believe that the feedback provider lacks the expertise to assess their performance
- A work or learning environment which does not explicitly value feedback and performance improvement

> Both receiving and providing feedback can be challenging; both skills can be developed and improved.

> Feedback has no effect in a vacuum; it must be linked to the situation and context by providing specific details.

Rationale: Why make the effort to provide constructive feedback?

Despite the challenges that providing feedback presents, learners need feedback on their learning and clinical performance from someone more expert, to know what they are doing well and what they need to improve. Without feedback, learners will not know how they are doing; they will learn more slowly and rely on poorly informed feedback from their peers or others less skilled. Ultimately, without feedback learners may harm patients.

Feedback informs learners' self-assessments, that is, their perceptions of how they are performing. We all need feedback to provide us with a realistic view of how we are doing. Without informed external feedback, our self-assessments can be unrealistic and even downright inaccurate.

Finally, as teachers and supervisors, feedback is one of our responsibilities to learners. Learners learn to practise medicine through experiential learning; that is, they learn by 'doing'. But it is not simply by 'doing' – it is through a cycle of 'doing', being observed by someone with expertise, receiving feedback from the expert on how to improve and 'doing' again.

Practice alone does **not** make perfect – it is practice with feedback that leads to improvement. Even those doing well can improve. Think of training to become a top athlete or musician; it is not just the practice that makes one excel, it is regular detailed feedback followed by more practice.

> Students and residents/registrars report rarely receiving feedback, and when they do, it is frequently too late or incomplete to be helpful.

What to do about it?

The following two sections provide suggestions for improving both the provision and reception of feedback.

> One goal for supervisors in providing feedback is to increase learners' comfort and skill in seeking, receiving and using feedback.

A shared definition of feedback can help

In clinical education, feedback is seen as 'specific information about the comparison between a trainee's observed performance and a standard, given with the intent to improve trainee's performance.' (van de Ridder *et al.* 2008). There are several useful points in this definition that can guide us:

- Provide **specific information**, not generalisations; for example, 'When you were describing the procedure to Mr Brown you used simple, non-medical language. He appeared to understand. A suggestion for next time is to also ask him if he understands.' This gives more useful information for the learner than just saying, 'You did well.'
- Feedback should be a **comparison between a trainee's observed performance and a standard**. Take time to observe your learner's performance. Share your observation with the learner along with the standard you are using or your rationale for the feedback you are giving; for example, 'I've found that the suturing goes more smoothly if I hold the forceps like this.'
- Feedback is '**given with the intent to improve trainees' performance**', rather than to criticise or judge. Viewing it this way can lessen anxiety around providing feedback and can help to focus on the features of feedback which enable learners to receive and use it.

> Practice alone does not make perfect – it is practice **with** feedback.

LIBRARY
EDUCATION CENTRE
PRINCESS ROYAL HOSPITAL

1. Observation of performance (P)	2. The feedback conversation (P, R)	3. Use of feedback for learning and change (R)
Includes · observation · understanding appropriate performance standards for the level of learner	*Includes for each (P and R)* · meeting face-to-face · describing what occurred · assessing what occurred · reflective problem-solving for improvement	*Includes* · accepting feedback · understanding what to do and how to change

Figure 7.1 The process of providing feedback for improvement (P = provider, R = receiver).

Tips to improve feedback effectiveness: bridging the gap between giving and receiving feedback

Refer to Figure 7.1 for an illustration of the steps included in providing feedback for improvement. The steps include observing learners' performance to collect specific information, engaging in a feedback discussion with the learner about your observations and the learner's perceptions, and helping the learner to use the feedback for improvement.

In Figure 7.2, we provide a simple feedback framework comprised of the following three critical components:

- Context and culture within which the feedback is provided
- Feedback provider
- Feedback receiver

Teachers and supervisors, as feedback providers, have responsibilities for each component.

Context and culture within which the feedback is provided

The **goal** is to create a 'culture of improvement' within your clinical workplace where sharing feedback is the norm, improvement is expected and feedback to guide that improvement is required. Such a culture makes giving feedback a routine aspect of work and learning. It makes it easier. It also models good practice for learners.

The following are the tips for creating a culture of improvement:

- Recognise that we as practitioners and supervisors also need to receive feedback to improve and learn.
- Ask for and attend to feedback from your learners and colleagues, and model this process for learners.
- Inform learners that you expect them to ask for feedback.
- Make giving and asking for feedback a routine learning activity; for example, schedule a few minutes each day, use a daily feedback form.
- Talk to medical and health profession colleagues about strategies for more openly sharing feedback with each other and learners.

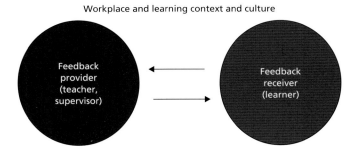

Workplace and learning context and culture

Feedback provider (teacher, supervisor)

Feedback receiver (learner)

Figure 7.2 A feedback framework: three critical components.

The feedback provider

Our **goal** as feedback providers is to increase both our comfort and skill in providing constructive feedback.

- View feedback as a positive activity to improve learners' performance and their self-assessment skills. View feedback as a routine expectation.
- Recognise that providing feedback is a skill which can be learnt and improved.
- Observe your learners in patient care to provide you with concrete data to use in feedback. Make time regularly for observation and feedback.
- Use effective feedback skills which guide learner improvement:
  ○ Be timely – as soon after your observation as possible. It only takes a few minutes.
  ○ Be specific not general, descriptive not judgemental; for example, 'I noticed that when you were counselling her about her medications, you read directly from your notes and did not make eye contact', not 'that was terrible.'
- Participate in activities to enhance your feedback skills; for example, attend development workshops, observe others providing feedback.

The feedback receiver

The **goal** for feedback providers is to increase learners' comfort and skill in seeking, receiving and using feedback. While learners may see the need for feedback to enable improvement, tension often exists between wanting to hear how one is doing and fearing that one is not measuring up.

- Identify feedback for your learners – before beginning, tell them you are giving them feedback.
- Consider the feedback encounter as a conversation between you and the learner, with improvement as the goal.
- Before providing your feedback, ask learners how they would assess their own performance. Encourage them to be specific and not use generalities like, 'I guess I did OK'.
- Before telling learners how to improve, engage them in reflective problem-solving about how they might improve and their goals.
- Some learners may need assistance in using their feedback; be prepared to provide helpful tips and give specific examples.
- Recognise that receiving feedback can be emotional.
  ○ Acknowledge that negative feedback can be disappointing, even a shock; for example, 'I know this is disappointing for you' or 'we all tend to feel angry when something like this surprises us'.
  ○ Acknowledge that emotional reactions are normal. Discussing them helps the learner to assimilate them, move on and look to improvement.
  ○ Stress that the purpose of feedback is not fault-finding but improving performance.

The most effective feedback is receiving information about a task and how to do it better; the least effective is related to praise, rewards and punishments.

— Hattie and Timperley, (2007)

Summary

In summary, while providing constructive feedback can be challenging, it is a skill which can be developed and improved. The benefits are substantial. Providing feedback effectively can markedly enhance your learners' learning and performance and increase your satisfaction as a supervisor and teacher.

Further reading

Cantillon P, Sargeant J. Teaching rounds: giving feedback in clinical settings. *BMJ* 2008;337(a1961):1292–1294.

Chowdhury RR, Kalu G. Learning to give feedback in medical education. *The Obstetrician & Gynaecologist* 2004;6:243–247.

Dudek NL, Marks MB. Failure to fail: the perspectives of clinical supervisors. *Academic Medicine* 2005;80(10):S84–S87.

References

Hattie J, Timperley H. The power of feedback. *Review of Educational Research* 2007 03/01;77(1):81–112.

van de Ridder JM, Stokking KM, McGaghie WC, ten Cate OT. What is feedback in clinical education? *Medical Education* 2008 Feb;42(2): 189–197.

CHAPTER 8

Learning and Teaching in the Clinical Environment

John Spencer

Newcastle University, Newcastle, UK

> **OVERVIEW**
>
> - The clinical setting has great potential as a learning environment, but there are many challenges
> - Effective clinical teachers know their subject, but they should also know about learning, their students and the curriculum
> - Learners need to be active participants; challenged but supported, and receive feedback
> - Patients can be actively involved and are generally pleased to help, but should be properly consented and their confidentiality should be maintained

Clinical education – that is, learning and teaching focused on, and involving, patients and their problems – lies at the heart of medical education. Medical schools strive to give students as much clinical exposure as possible, increasingly from early in the curriculum. For postgraduates, 'on-the-job' clinical teaching is at the core of their professional development. So, how can clinical teachers optimise the teaching and learning opportunities that arise in daily practice?

Strengths, problems and challenges of clinical education

Learning in the clinical environment has many strengths. It is focused on real problems in the workplace. Learners are motivated by its obvious relevance and through active participation, particularly when they feel they are contributing to patient care; their confidence and enthusiasm are boosted. It is the only setting in which the full array of technical and non-technical skills, attitudes and applied knowledge that constitute 'doctoring' are 'modelled' by clinical teachers. Essential attributes such as history taking and examination, clinical reasoning, appraising risk, managing uncertainty, explanation, planning and decision-making, record keeping, teamworking and leadership can all be learnt as an integrated whole. Despite these potential strengths, clinical education has been much criticised for its variability, lack of intellectual

challenge and haphazard nature. In the words of one author, it is 'a conceptually sound model, flawed by problems of implementation' (Box 8.1). Clinical teachers also face many challenges in their work; some go with the job, but many can be tackled with careful planning (Box 8.2).

> Box 8.1 **Common problems with clinical teaching**
>
> - Lack of clear objectives or expectations
> - Focus on factual recall rather than reasoning and skills
> - Teaching pitched at wrong level
> - Learners not actively involved
> - Inadequate supervision and lack of feedback
> - Little opportunity for reflection
> - Teaching by humiliation
> - Patients not properly consented
> - Lack of respect for dignity of patient
> - Lack of congruence or continuity with rest of the curriculum

> Box 8.2 **Challenges of clinical teaching**
>
> **Environment**
> - Physical environment not 'teaching friendly'
> - Requirements of infection control
> - Lack of space
>
> **Patients**
> - Fewer patients (unavailable; shorter hospital stays; too frail or sick)
> - Consent and confidentiality
>
> **Students**
> - Learners of different abilities and levels
> - Increased numbers
> - Not prepared for clinical learning
>
> **Teachers**
> - No training in teaching and learning
> - Unfamiliar with the curriculum
> - Not knowing the students
> - Poor rewards and recognition
> - Competing demands (patient care, administration, research, wanting a 'life')
> - Time pressures

ABC of Learning and Teaching in Medicine, 2nd edition.
Edited by Peter Cantillon and Diana Wood. © 2010 Blackwell Publishing Ltd.

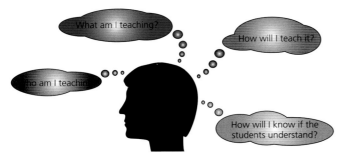

Figure 8.1 Questions to ask when planning a clinical teaching session.

Planning

The importance of planning cannot be overstated; indeed, preparation is recognised by students as evidence of a good clinical teacher. Far from compromising spontaneity, planning provides structure and context for both teachers and learners, as well as a framework for reflection and evaluation. At the very least, there are a few questions that you should ask yourself in advance of every teaching session (Figure 8.1).

How learners learn

Understanding something about learning will help clinical teachers be more effective. Several theories are relevant (see Chapter 1). All start with the premise that learning is an active process (and by inference that the teacher's role is to act as facilitator rather than font of all knowledge). Cognitive theories argue that learning involves processing information through interplay between existing knowledge and new knowledge. An important influencing factor is what the learner knows already. The quality of the resulting new knowledge depends not only on 'activating' this prior knowledge but also on the degree of restructuring or elaboration that takes place. The more elaborated the resulting knowledge is, the more easily it will be retrieved, particularly when learning takes place in the context in which the knowledge will be used (Box 8.3).

Box 8.3 **How to use cognitive learning theory in teaching**

Help learners identify what they already know

- Activate prior knowledge by brainstorming and briefing

Help learners restructure and elaborate their knowledge

- Provide a bridge between existing and new information, for example, use of clinical examples, analogies, comparisons
- Provide learners with opportunities to see how presentations of the same disease manifest in different ways from patient to patient
- Debrief learners afterwards
- Promote reflection

Experiential learning

Experiential learning theory holds that learning is a cyclical process linking concrete experience (practice) with abstract

---

Figure 8.2 Experiential learning cycle: the role of the teacher is to help students to complete the cycle.

conceptualisation (theory) through reflection and planning. Reflection involves standing back and thinking about experience (What did it mean? How does it relate to previous experience? How did I do and how did it feel?). Most students do not reflect spontaneously, so need help and guidance. Planning involves anticipating the application of new theories and skills (What will I do next time?). The learning cycle itself provides a useful framework for planning teaching sessions (Box 8.4 and Figure 8.2).

Box 8.4 **Example of using experiential learning cycle as framework for a clinical teaching session**

Setting: Small group of third year medical students on introductory clinical skills – placement in general practice
Topics: History taking and examination of patients with rheumatoid arthritis – two or three patients with good stories and signs recruited from the community
Planning: Brainstorm about presentation of rheumatoid arthritis (typical symptoms and signs) – this activates prior knowledge, orientates and provides a framework for the task
Experience: Students interview patients in pairs, and then carry out focused examination under supervision – provides opportunities for the so-called 'deliberate practice' and to receive feedback
Reflection: Case presentations, discussion of findings and feedback – provide opportunities for elaboration of learning
Theorising: Didactic input from teacher (or student) of a basic clinical overview of rheumatoid disease – helps link theory with practice
Planning: 'What have I learnt?' and 'What will I do differently next time?' – help prepare students for the next encounter, also enable evaluation of the session

---

How doctors teach

Almost all doctors are involved in clinical education at some point in their careers, and most undertake the job conscientiously and enthusiastically. However, few receive any formal training in teaching, and historically there was an assumption that if a person simply knew a lot about their subject, they could teach it. In reality, of course, although subject expertise is important, it is not sufficient. Effective clinical teachers actually use several distinct, if overlapping, forms of knowledge (Figure 8.3).

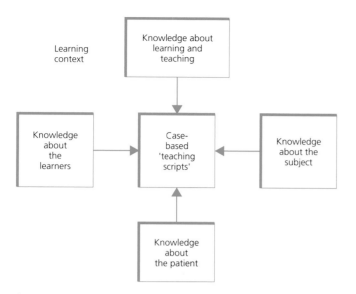

Figure 8.3 Knowledge domains used by effective clinical teachers to inform development of case-based teaching scripts.

Communication and teaching

Effective teaching depends crucially on the teacher's communication skills. Two key areas are asking questions and giving explanations. Both are underpinned by attentive listening and sensitivity to the learners' verbal and non-verbal cues.

Questioning

Questions may fulfil many purposes, for example, clarifying understanding, promoting curiosity, emphasising key points and diagnosing strengths and weaknesses. They can be classified as 'closed', 'open' and 'clarifying' (or 'probing') questions. Closed questions invoke relatively low-order thinking, often simple recall. Indeed, a closed question may elicit no response at all (for example, because the learner is worried about being wrong), and the teacher may end up answering his or her own question! In theory, open questions are more likely to promote deeper thinking, but if they are too broad they may be equally ineffective. The purpose of clarifying and probing questions is self-evident (Box 8.5).

> **Box 8.5 Questioning**
>
> Questioning can be pitched at three broad cognitive levels:
>
> - Recall – *What? Which? Where?*
> - Comprehension – *Why? How?*
> - Problem-solving – *What if?*

Explanation

Clinical teaching usually involves a lot of explanation, ranging from the (all too common) mini-lecture to 'thinking aloud'. The latter is a powerful way of 'modelling' professional thinking, giving the novice insight into experts' clinical reasoning and problem-solving (not easily articulated formally).

There are close analogies between teacher–student and doctor–patient communication, and the principles for giving clear explanations apply, namely: check understanding before, during and after the explanation; provide information in 'bite-size chunks'; summarise periodically and at the end (better still, ask one of the learners to summarise); highlight take-home messages; finally, invite questions. If in doubt, pitch things at a low level and work upwards. As the late Sydney Jacobson, a journalist, said, 'Never underestimate the person's intelligence, but don't overestimate their knowledge.' Feedback is a powerful influence on learning but is an underused strategy (see Chapter 7).

Exploiting teaching opportunities

Most clinical teaching takes place in the context of busy practice, with time at a premium. Many studies have shown that a disproportionate amount of time in teaching sessions may be spent on regurgitation of facts, with relatively little on checking, probing and developing understanding. Several models for using time more effectively and efficiently and integrating teaching into day-to-day routines have been described (Box 8.6).

> **Box 8.6 Tips for time-limited teaching**
>
> **Step 1 – Identify the learner's needs**
>
> - Ask questions – before the clinical encounter
> - Conduct a 2-minute observation of the learner – followed by brief discussion
>
> **Step 2 – Select a model for time-limited teaching**
>
> - The 'one-minute preceptor' model (see Figure 8.4)
> - The 'Aunt Minnie' model – pattern recognition and focused discussion
> - Student makes specific observations – discussion at end
> - 'Hot-seating' – for all or part of the consultation
>
> **Step 3 – Provide feedback**
>
> - Encourage self-evaluation
> - Focus on strengths and specific areas for improvement

Teaching on the wards

Despite a long and worthy tradition, the hospital ward is not an ideal teaching venue. Nonetheless, with preparation and forethought, learning opportunities can be maximised with minimal disruption to staff, patients and relatives. Approaches include teaching on ward rounds (either special teaching rounds or during 'business' rounds, with or without pre- and post-round meetings); dedicated sessions with selected patients; students seeing patients on their own (or in pairs – students can learn a lot from each other) and then reporting back, with or without a follow-up visit to the bedside for further discussion; and shadowing, when learning will

LIBRARY
EDUCATION CENTRE
PRINCESS ROYAL HOSPITAL

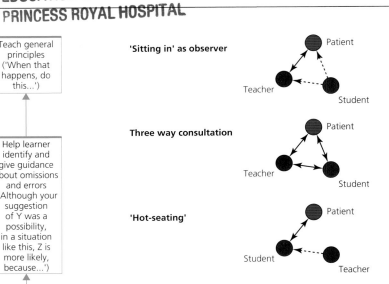

Patient encounter (history, examination, etc)

Get a commitment ('What do you think is going on?')

Probe for underlying reasoning ('What led you to that conclusion?')

Teach general principles ('When that happens, do this...')

Help learner identify and give guidance about omissions and errors ('Although your suggestion of Y was a possibility, in a situation like this, Z is more likely, because...')

Reinforce what was done well ('Your diagnosis of X was well supported by the history...')

Figure 8.4 'One-minute preceptor' model.

'Sitting in' as observer — Patient, Teacher, Student

Three way consultation — Patient, Teacher, Student

'Hot-seating' — Patient, Student, Teacher

Figure 8.5 Seating arrangements for teaching in ambulatory clinics.

inevitably be opportunistic. Key issues are careful selection of patients; ensuring ward staff know what is happening; briefing patients as well as students; using a side room (rather than the bedside) for further discussions about patients; and ensuring that all relevant information (such as records and X-ray images) is available.

Teaching in the ambulatory clinic

Although teaching during consultations in ambulatory clinics (i.e. out patients or general practice) has great potential, it is limited in what it can achieve if students remain only passive observers. However, with relatively little impact on the running of a clinic, students can participate more actively. For example, they can make specific observations, write down thoughts about differential diagnosis or further tests, or note any questions – for discussion with the teacher in between patients. A more active approach is 'hot-seating'. Here the student leads the consultation, or part of it. Their findings can be checked with the patient, and discussion and feedback can take place during or after the encounter. Students, although daunted, find this rewarding. A third model is when a student sees a patient alone, and is then joined by the tutor. The student then presents their findings, and discussion follows. A limitation is that the teacher does not see the student in action. It also inevitably slows the clinic down, although not as much as might be expected. There are several other ways of organising a clinic according to purpose, number of students and so on. In an ideal world, it is always sensible to block out time in a clinic to accommodate teaching (Figure 8.5).

The patient's role

Sir William Osler's dictum that 'it is a safe rule to have no teaching without a patient for a text, and the best teaching is that taught by the patient himself' is well known. The importance of learning from the patient has been repeatedly emphasised. For example, generations of students have been exhorted to 'listen to the patient – he is telling you the diagnosis.' Traditionally, however, the role has been essentially passive, the patient acting as interesting teaching material, often no more than a medium through which the teacher teaches. Apart from being potentially disrespectful, this is a wasted opportunity. Not only can patients tell their stories and demonstrate physical signs but they can also give deeper and broader insights into their problems. Finally, they can give feedback to both learners and teacher. Through their interactions with patients, clinical teachers – knowingly or unknowingly – have a powerful influence on learners as role models (Box 8.7).

Box 8.7 **Working effectively and ethically with patients**

- Think about which parts of the session require direct patient contact – is it necessary to have a discussion at the bedside?
- Obtain consent before learners arrive (or at least before the patient enters the consulting room!)
- Ensure students respect confidentiality of all information relating to the patient – verbal, written or electronic
- Brief the patient before the encounter – purpose of the session, level of learners' experience, what is expected of the patient, any concerns?
- If appropriate, actively involve the patient in the teaching – use their expertise
- Ask the patient for feedback – about communication skills, attitudes and bedside manner
- Debrief the patient after the encounter – he or she may have questions, or sensitive issues may have been raised

Further reading

Cox K. Planning bedside teaching. (Parts 1 to 8.) *The Medical Journal of Australia* 1993;158:280–282, 355–357, 417–418, 493–495, 571–572, 607–608, 789–790, and 159:64–65.

Dornan T, Scherpbier A, Boshuizen H. Supporting medical students' workplace learning. Experience-based learning. *The Clinical Teacher* 2009;6: 167–171.

Hargreaves DH, Southworth GW, Stanley P, Ward SJ. *On-the-job Learning for Physicians.* London: Royal Society of Medicine, 1997.

Irby DM, Wilkerson L. Teaching when time is limited. *BMJ* 2008;336: 384–387.

Reilly B. Inconvenient truths about effective clinical teaching. *The Lancet* 2007;370(9588):705–711.

Sprake C, Cantillon P, Metcalf J, Spencer J. Teaching in an ambulatory care setting. *BMJ* 2008;337:690–692.

CHAPTER 9

Written Assessment

Lambert W T Schuwirth and Cees P M van der Vleuten

Maastricht University, Maastricht, The Netherlands

OVERVIEW

- Choosing the most appropriate type of written examination for a certain purpose is often difficult
- Some knowledge cannot be tested with multiple-choice questions, and some knowledge is best not tested with open-ended questions
- The five criteria – reliability, validity, educational impact, cost-effectiveness and acceptability – are helpful in evaluating the advantages and disadvantages of various question types

---

Many misconceptions still exist about written assessment, despite being disproved repeatedly by scientific studies. Probably, the most important misconception is the belief that the format of the question plays an important role in determining what the question actually tests. Multiple-choice questions, for example, are often believed to be unsuitable for testing medical problem-solving. The reasoning behind this assumption is that all a student has to do in a multiple-choice question is to recognise the correct answer, whereas, in an open-ended question he/she has to generate the answer spontaneously. However, research has repeatedly shown that the question's format is of limited importance and that it is the content of the question that determines almost totally what the question tests.

This does not imply that question formats are always interchangeable – some knowledge cannot be tested with multiple-choice questions, and some knowledge is best not tested with open-ended questions.

If one wants to evaluate the advantages and disadvantages of various question types, the five criteria – reliability, validity, educational impact, cost-effectiveness and acceptability – are helpful.

Reliability pertains to the accuracy with which a score on a test is determined (Box 9.1).

Validity refers to whether the question actually tests what it is purported to test (Box 9.2).

Educational impact is important because students tend to focus strongly on what they believe will be in the examinations and they will prepare strategically depending on the question types used.

ABC of Learning and Teaching in Medicine, 2nd edition.
Edited by Peter Cantillon and Diana Wood. © 2010 Blackwell Publishing Ltd.

Box 9.1 **Reliability**

- A score that a student obtains on a test should indicate the score that this student would obtain in any other given (equally difficult) test in the same field ('parallel test').
- A test represents at best a sample selected from the domain of all applicable and relevant questions. So, if a student passes a particular test one has to be sure that he/she would not have failed a parallel test, and vice versa.
- The following two factors influence reliability negatively:
  - The number of items may be too small to provide a reproducible result or the questions focus only on a certain element, so the scores cannot generalise to the whole discipline.
  - The items may be poorly produced, ambiguous or difficult to read, thus leading to a false negative or false positive response.

Box 9.2 **Validity**

- The validity of a test is the extent to which it measures what it purports to measure.
- Most competencies cannot be observed directly (body length, for example, can be observed directly; intelligence has to be derived from observations). Therefore, in examinations it is important to collect evidence to ensure validity:
  - *One simple piece* of evidence could be, for example, that experts score higher than students on the test.
  - *Alternative approaches* include (i) an analysis of the distribution of course topics within test elements (a so called blueprint) and (ii) an assessment of the soundness of individual test items.
- Good validation of tests should use several different pieces of evidence.

Whether different preparation leads to different types of knowledge is not fully clear, however. When teachers are forced to use a particular question type, they will tend to ask about the themes that can be easily assessed with that question type, and they will neglect the topics for which the question type is less well suited. Therefore, it is wise to vary the question types in different examinations.

Cost-effectiveness and acceptability are important as the costs of different examinations have to be taken into account, and even the best designed examination will not survive if it is not accepted by teachers and students.

Written formats not to be used

Although, virtually all assessment methods have strengths and weaknesses, there are some formats in which the disadvantages outweigh the advantages so strongly that it is best not to use them at all. This is mainly true for complicated multiple-choice questions. One of these typically presents the candidates with four or five statements and the candidates have to select the combination of correct statements from the options. An example is provided in Box 9.3.

Box 9.3 **Complicated multiple-choice question**

Morphine as a drug in the treatment of severe pain

1. is addictive to all patients who use it
2. can lead to constipation
3. can lead to nausea and vomiting
4. has COX-inhibition as its main mechanism of action

a. 1, 2 and 3 are correct
b. 2 and 3 are correct
c. 1, 3 and 4 are correct
d. all are correct

Another format consists of two statements combined with a conjunction. The candidates then have to determine the correctness of the statements and the conjunction. None of these formats test medical knowledge or reasoning better, they only complicate matters.

True or false questions

The main advantage of 'true or false questions' is their conciseness (Box 9.4). A question can be answered quickly by the student, so the test can cover a broad domain. Such questions have two major disadvantages. Firstly, they are difficult to construct flawlessly – the statements have to be defensibly true or absolutely false. Secondly, when a student answers a 'false' question correctly, we can conclude only that the student knew the statement was false, not that he/she knew the correct fact. Because of these major problems it is best to avoid using them or to replace them by single, best option multiple-choice items.

Box 9.4 **True or false questions**

True or false questions are most suitable when the purpose of the question is to test whether students are able to evaluate the correctness of an assumption; in other cases, they are best avoided.

'Single, best option' multiple-choice questions

Multiple-choice questions are well known, and there is extensive experience worldwide in constructing them (Box 9.5). Their main advantage is the high reliability per hour of testing. This is mainly because they can be answered quickly and thus a broad domain can be covered in a short space of time. They are often easier to construct than true or false questions and are more versatile. If properly constructed, multiple-choice questions can test more than simple facts but unfortunately they are often only used to test facts, as teachers often think this is all they are fit for. A useful guide to their construction can be found on the website of the National Board of Medical Examiners (http://www.nbme.org/publications/item-writing-manual.html).

Box 9.5 **Multiple-choice questions**

Multiple-choice questions can be used in many forms of testing, except when spontaneous generation of the answer is essential, such as in creativity, hypothesising and writing skills. Teachers need to be taught how to write good multiple-choice questions.

Multiple true or false questions

This format enables the teacher to ask a question to which there is more than one correct answer (Box 9.6). Although they take somewhat longer to answer than the previous two types, their reliability per hour of testing time is not much lower.

Box 9.6 **Multiple true or false questions**

Which of the following drugs belong to the ACE inhibitor group?

a. atenolol	**h.** metoprolol
b. pindolol	**i.** propranolol
c. amiloride	**j.** triamterene
d. furosemide	**k.** captopril
e. enalapril	**l.** verapamil
f. clopamide	**m.** digoxin
g. epoprostenol	

Construction, however, is not easy. It is important to have sufficient distracters (incorrect options) and to find a good balance between the number of correct options and distracters.

In addition, it is essential to construct the question so that correct options are defensibly correct and distracters are defensibly incorrect. A further disadvantage is the rather complicated scoring procedure for these questions.

'Short answer' open-ended questions

Open-ended questions are more flexible in that they can test issues that require, for example, creativity and spontaneity, but they have lower reliability per hour of testing time (Box 9.7). Answering open-ended questions is much more time consuming than answering multiple-choice questions so they are less suitable for broad sampling. They are also expensive to produce and to score. When writing open-ended questions it is important to describe clearly how detailed the answer should be – without giving away the answer. A good open-ended question should include a detailed model answer key for the person marking the paper. Short answer, open-ended questions are not suitable for assessing factual knowledge; use multiple-choice questions instead.

Box 9.7 **Open-ended question**

Open-ended questions are perhaps the most widely accepted question type. Their format is commonly believed to be intrinsically superior to a multiple-choice format. Much evidence shows, however, that this assumed superiority is limited.

Short answer, open-ended questions should be aimed at the aspects of competence that cannot be tested in any other way.

Essays

Essays are ideal for assessing how well students can summarise, hypothesise, find relationships and apply known procedures to new situations. They can also provide an insight into different aspects of writing ability and the ability to process information.

Unfortunately, using the essay format to answer questions is time consuming.

When constructing essay questions, it is essential to define the criteria on which the answers will be judged. A common pitfall is to 'over-structure' these criteria in the pursuit of objectivity and this often leads to trivialisation of the questions. Some structure and criteria are necessary, but too detailed a structure provides little gain in reliability and a considerable loss of validity. Essays involve high costs, so they should be used sparsely and only in cases where short answer, open-ended questions or multiple-choice questions are not appropriate.

'Key feature' questions

A key feature question consists of a realistic description of a case followed by a small number of questions aimed at the essential decisions for the problem-solving process (Box 9.8). The questions may be either multiple choice or open ended, depending on the content of the question. Key feature questions are a valid measurement of problem-solving ability and have good reliability. In addition, most people involved in setting and marking them consider them to be suitable, which makes them more acceptable.

The key feature format is new and therefore less well known than the other approaches. Construction of the questions is time consuming; inexperienced teachers may need up to 3 hours to produce a single key feature case with questions. Experienced writers, though, may produce up to four an hour. Nevertheless, these questions are expensive to produce, and large numbers of cases are normally needed to produce a reasonable bank. Key feature questions are best used for testing the application of knowledge and problem-solving in 'high stakes' examinations.

Box 9.8 **Example of a key feature question**

Case

You are a general practitioner. Yesterday you made a house call on Mr Downing. From your history taking and physical examination you diagnosed nephrolithiasis. You gave an intramuscular injection of 100 mg diclofenac, and you left him some diclofenac suppositories. You advised him to take one when in pain but not more than two a day. Today he rings you at 9 am. He still has pain attacks, which respond well to the diclofenac, but since 5 am he has also had continuous pain in his right side and fever (38.9°C).

Which of the following is the best next step?

a. Ask him to wait another day to see how the disease progresses.
b. Prescribe broad-spectrum antibiotics.
c. Refer him to hospital for an intravenous pyelogram.
d. Refer him urgently to a urologist.

Extended matching questions

The key elements of extended matching questions (EMQs) are a list of options, a 'lead-in' question and some case descriptions or vignettes (Box 9.9). Students should understand that an option may be correct for more than one vignette and some options may not apply to any of the vignettes. The idea is to minimise the cueing effect that occurs in standard MCQs because of the many possible combinations between vignettes and options. Also, by using cases instead of facts, the items can be used to test application of knowledge or problem-solving ability. They are easier to construct than key feature questions as many cases can be derived from one set of options. Their reliability has been shown to

---

Box 9.9 **Example of an extended matching question**

a. *Campylobacter jejuni*	**i.** *Helicobacter pylori*
b. *Candida albicans*	**j.** *Clostridium perfringens*
c. *Giardia lamblia*	**k.** *Mycobacterium tuberculosis*
d. *Rotavirus*	**l.** *Shigella flexneri*
e. *Salmonella typhi*	**m.** *Vibrio cholerae*
f. *Yersinia enterocolitica*	**n.** *Clostridium difficile*
g. *Pseudomonas aeruginosa*	**o.** *Proteus mirabilis*
h. *Escherichia coli*	**p.** *Tropheryma whippelii*

For each of the following cases, select (from the list above) the microorganism most likely to be responsible:

- A 48-year-old man with a chronic complaint of dyspepsia suddenly develops severe abdominal pain. On physical examination there is general tenderness to palpation with rigidity and rebound tenderness. Abdominal radiography shows free air under the diaphragm.
- A 45-year-old woman is treated with antibiotics for recurring respiratory tract infections. She develops a severe abdominal pain with haemorrhagic diarrhoea. Endoscopically a pseudomembranous colitis is seen.

be good and they are now in widespread use. Scoring of the answers is easy and can be done by computer.

Teachers need training and practice before they can write EMQs and there is a risk of an under-representation of certain themes simply because they do not fit the format. EMQs are best used when large numbers of similar sorts of decisions (for example, relating to diagnosis or ordering of laboratory tests) need testing for different situations.

Script-concordance test

A final format to consider is the script-concordance test (Box 9.10). In this format, a very brief scenario is presented to the candidates with a hypothesis about a diagnosis. The candidates are then asked to indicate the value of certain symptoms or findings for diagnosis. An example is given in Box 9.10. Script-concordance tests are developed to assess the degree of concordance between the candidate and experts in the way their knowledge – essential for successful problem-solving – is organised in their memories. The scoring is based on the amount of agreement between the candidate and the experts. The concept is firmly based in the current theories on medical expertise and various studies have shown reliability and indications of validity. Apart from being a rather new and

---

Box 9.10 **Script-concordance test**

A 24-year-old woman presents at the emergency with acute severe abdominal pain in the right lower quadrant.

If you are thinking of an ectopic pregnancy and the patient reports that she is using an intrauterine contraceptive device, the hypothesis becomes:

−3 Ruled out
−2 Much less probable
−1 A little less probable
  0 No effect on this hypothesis
  1 A little more probable
  2 Much more probable
  3 Certain

---

possibly unfamiliar method, it also requires careful selection of the specific questions for the cases. They need to be aimed at critical deliberations in the problem-solving process. Also, as there is no prefixed answer key, a panel of experts is needed to provide a reference for the scoring.

Conclusion

Choosing the best question type for a particular examination is not simple. A careful balancing of costs and benefits is required. A well-designed assessment programme will use different types of question appropriate for the content being tested (Box 9.11). This chapter can only provide a brief introduction and for a more detailed explanation of the dos and don'ts of each question format it is wise to consult more detailed texts.

Box 9.11 **Conclusion**

Using only one type of question throughout the whole curriculum is not a valid approach.

Further reading

Case SM, Swanson DB. Extended-matching items: a practical alternative to free response questions. *Teaching and Learning in Medicine* 1993;5: 107–115.

Charlin B, Brailovsky C, Leduc C, Blouin D. The diagnostic script questionnaire: a new tool to assess a specific dimension of clinical competence. *Advances in Health Science Education* 1998;3:51–58.

Page G, Bordage G. The Medical Council of Canada's key features project: a more valid written examination of clinical decision-making skills. *Academic Medicine* 1995;70(2):104–110.

Schuwirth LWT, Blackmore DB, Mom E, Van de Wildenberg F, Stoffers H, Van der Vleuten CPM. How to write short cases for assessing problem-solving skills. *Medical Teacher* 1999;21(2):144–150.

Swanson DB, Norcini JJ, Grosso LJ. Assessment of clinical competence: written and computer-based simulations. *Assessment and Evaluation in Higher Education* 1987;12:220–246.

CHAPTER 10

Skill-Based Assessment

Val Wass

Keele University, Keele, UK

OVERVIEW

- To understand the place of skill-based assessment in testing methodology
- To apply basic assessment principles to skill-based assessment
- To plan the content of a skill-based assessment
- To design a skill-based assessment
- To understand the advantages and disadvantages of skill-based assessment

Background

Medical educators must ensure that health professionals, throughout training, are safe to work with patients. This requires integration of knowledge, skills and professional behaviour. Miller's triangle (Figure 10.1) offers a useful framework for understanding the assessment of competency across developing clinical expertise. Analogies are often made with the airline industry where simulation ('shows how') is heavily relied upon. Medicine is moving away from simulation to test what a doctor actually 'does' in the workplace-based assessment (WPBA) (Chapter 11). For logistical reasons, the WPBA methodology still lacks the high reliability needed to guarantee safety. Simulated demonstration ('shows how') of effective integration of written knowledge (Chapter 9) into practice remains essential to assure competent clinical performance.

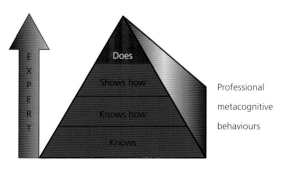

Figure 10.1 Miller's triangle (adapted) as a model for competency testing.

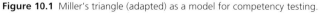

ABC of Learning and Teaching in Medicine, 2nd edition.
Edited by Peter Cantillon and Diana Wood. © 2010 Blackwell Publishing Ltd.

This chapter offers a framework for the design and delivery of skill-based assessments (SBAs).

Applying basic assessment principles to skill-based assessment (SBA):

Basic assessment principles must be applied when designing the SBA (Wass *et al*. 2001). Table 10.1 defines these key concepts and their relevance to SBA.

Summative versus formative

The purpose of the SBA must be clearly defined and transparent to candidates. With increasing development of WPBA, skill

Table 10.1 The assessment of clinical skills: key issues when planning.

Definition of key concepts	Relevance to SBA
Formative/summative Summative tests involve potentially threatening high-stakes pass/fail judgements. Formative tests give constructive feedback	Clarify the purpose of the test. Offer formative opportunities wherever possible
Context specificity A skill is bound in the context in which it is performed	Professionals perform inconsistently. Sample widely across different contexts
Blue printing A test must be mapped against curriculum learning outcomes	Only include competencies which cannot be more efficiently tested elsewhere
Reliability 'The degree to which a test is consistent and reproducible'. A 100% consistency equates quantitatively with a coefficient score of 1.0.	Sample adequately. Test length is crucial. Use a range of contexts and different assessors
Validity 'The degree to which a test has measured what it set out to measure'. A conceptual term; difficult to quantify	Has the SBA been true to the blueprint and tested integrated practical skills?
Standard setting Define the criterion standard of 'minimum competency' i.e. the pass/fail cut-off score	Use robust, defensible, internationally accepted methodology

Wass *et al*. 2001.

GP Postgraduate OSCE Blueprint	Primary nature of case					
Primary system or area of disease	Acute	Chronic	Undiffer entiated	Psycho /Social	Prevention /Lifestyle	Other
Cardiovascular	1					
Respiratory		2				
Neurological/ Psychiatric				9		
Musculo-skeletal	12					
Endocrine & Oncological			13	11		
Eye/ENT/Skin	8		3			
Men's/Women's Sexual Health					4	10
Renal/Urologcal	6					
Gastro-intestinal			7			
Infectious diseases					5	14
Other						

Key: ▨ represents an individual station as placed on the grid numbered 1–14.

Figure 10.2 An example blueprint of a SBA mapping 14 ten-minute doctor–patient interactions.

assessment per se often takes a 'summative' function focused on reliably assessing minimal competency, that is, whether the trainee is considered 'safe' to progress to the next stage of training or not. From the public's perspective, this is a 'high-stakes' summative decision. Candidates may have potentially conflicting expectations for 'formative' feedback on their performance. Opportunities to give this, either directly or through breakdown of results, should be built in wherever possible. SBAs are high resource tests. Optimising their educational advantage is essential.

Blueprinting

SBAs must be mapped to curriculum learning outcomes. This is termed *blueprinting*. The test should be interactive and assess skills which cannot be assessed using less highly resourced methods. For example, the interpretation of data and images is more efficiently tested in written or electronic format. Similarly, the blueprint should assign skills best tested 'on-the-job', for example, management of acutely ill patients, to WPBA. Figure 10.2 is a blueprint of a postgraduate SBA in general practice where skills (horizontal axis) relevant to primary care, for example, 'undifferentiated presentations', can be mapped against the context of different specialties (vertical axis).

Context specificity

Professionals perform inconsistently across tasks. Context specificity is not unique to medicine. It reflects the way professionals learn experientially and inconsistently (Box 10.1). Thus they perform well in some domains and less well in others. Understanding this concept is intrinsic and essential to assessment design. Performance on one problem does not predict performance on another. This applies equally to skills such as communication and professionalism, sometimes wrongly perceived as generic. The knowledge and environment, that is, context, in which the skill is performed cannot be divorced from the skill itself.

Box 10.1 **Context specificity**

- Professionals perform inconsistently across tasks.
- We are all good at some things and less good at others.
- Wide sampling in different contexts is essential.

Blueprinting is essential. It is very easy to collate questions set in similar rather than contrasting contexts. This undergraduate blueprint (Figure 10.3) will not test students across a range of

Skills	Context/domain										
	CVS	Respiratory	Abdomen	CNS	Joints	Eyes	ENT	GUM	Mental state	Skin	Endocrine
History taking	Heart failure			Epilepsy							New diabetic
Physical exam	Heart murmur		Mass	Cranial nerves	Back					Rash eczema	Diabetic foot
Communication	Post MI Advice										Explaining insulin
Clinical procedures	Iv cann-ulation	Resuscitation								Suturing	Blood glucose

Figure 10.3 14-station undergraduate OSCE which fails to address context specificity. The four skill areas being tested (history taking, physical examination, communication and clinical procedures) are mapped according to the domain speciality or context in which they are set to ensure that a full range of curriculum content is covered.

contexts. The focus is, probably quite inadvertently, on cardio-vascular and diabetes. Careful planning is essential to optimise sampling across all curriculum domains.

Reliability

Reliability is a quantitative measure applied both to the repro-ducibility of a test (inter-case reliability) and the consistency of assessor ratings (inter-rater reliability) (Downing 2004). For both measurements, theoretically, achieving 100% reliability gives a coef-ficient of 1. In reality, high stakes skill assessments should aim to achieve coefficients greater than 0.8.

Adequate sampling across the curriculum blueprint is essential to reliably assess a candidate's ability by addressing context specificity. Figure 10.4 offers statistical guidance on the number of stations required. Above 14 will give sufficient reliability for a high stakes test. Inter-rater reliability is such that one examiner per station suffices.

A SBA rarely achieves reliabilities greater than 0.8. It proves impossible to minimise factors adversely affecting reproducibility – for example, standardisation of simulations and assessor inconsis-tencies. These factors must be minimised through careful planning, training assessors and simulators and so on (Table 10.2).

Validity

Validity is a difficult conceptual term (Hodges 2003) and a challenge for SBA design. Many argue that taking 'snapshots' of candidates' abilities, as SBAs tend to do, is inadequate. Validity can only be evaluated by retrospectively reviewing SBA content and test scores to ascertain whether they accurately reflect the curriculum at an appropriate level of expertise. For example, if a normal subject is substituted on a varicose vein examination station when a scheduled patient cancels, the station loses its validity.

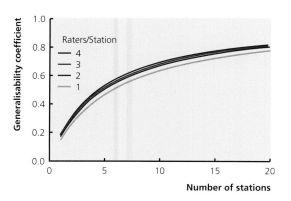

Figure 10.4 Statistics demonstrating how reliability (generalisability coefficient) improves as station number is increased and the number of raters on each station is increased. (Figure reproduced with kind permission from Dave Swanson, using data from Newble DI, Swanson DB. Psychometric characteristics of the objective structured clinical examination. *Medical Education* 1988;22:325–334 and Swanson DB, Clauser BE, Case SM. Clinical skills assessment with standardised patients in high-stakes tests: a framework for thinking about score precision, equating, and security. *Advances in Health Sciences Education* 1999;4:67–106.)

Table 10.2 Measures for improving reliability.

Factor	Measure
Inadequate sampling	Monitor reliability. Increase stations if unsatisfactory
Station content	Ask examiners and SPs to evaluate stations. Check performance statistics[a]
Confused candidates	Process must be transparent, brief them on the day and make station instructions short and task focused
Erratic examiners	Examiner selection and training is absolutely essential
Inconsistent role play	Ensure scenarios are detailed and SPs trained. Monitor performance across circuits
Real patient logistics	Reserves are essential
Fatigue and dehydration	Comfort breaks and refreshments mandatory
Noise level	Ensure circuits have adequate space. Monitor noise level
Poor administration	Use staff who can multitask and attend to detail

[a]The SPSS package analyses reliability with individual station item removed. If reliability improves without the station, it is seriously flawed.

Standard setting

In high-stakes testing, transparent, criterion-referenced pass/fail cut-off scores must be set using established and defensible method-ology. Historically 'norm referencing', that is, passing a predeter-mined number of the candidate cohort, was used. This is no longer acceptable. Various methods are available to agree on the standard before (Angoff, Ebel), during (Borderline Regression) and after (Hofstee) the test (Norcini 2003). We lack a gold standard method-ology. Use more than one method where possible. Pre-set standards tend to be too high and may need adjustment. Above all, the cut-off score must be defined by those familiar with the curriculum and candidates. Informed, realistic judgements are essential.

Agreeing on the content

Confusion is emerging as SBAs assume different titles: Objective Structured Clinical Examination (OSCE), Clinical Skills Assessment (CSA), Simulated Surgeries, PACES and so on. The principles outlined above apply to all formats. The design and structure of circuits varies according to the needs of the speciality.

Designing the circuit

Figure 10.5 outlines a basic structure for a 14-station SBA. The con-tent and length of stations can vary provided the constructs being tested, for example, communication and examination skills, sample widely across the blueprinted contexts. The plan should include rest periods for candidates, examiners and simulated patients (SPs). Fatigue adversely affects performance. In most tests the candi-date circulates (Figure 10.6). Variances can occur; in the MRCGP 'simulated surgery' the candidate remains static while the SP and examiner move. Station length can vary, even within the assessment, according to the time needed to perform the skill and level of exper-tise under test. The design should maximise the validity of the assess-ment. Inevitably, a compromise is needed to balance reliability, validity, logistics and resource restraints. If the SBA is formative and

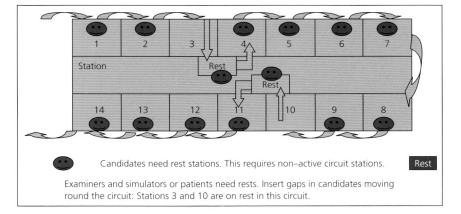

Candidates need rest stations. This requires non–active circuit stations.

Rest

Examiners and simulators or patients need rests. Insert gaps in candidates moving round the circuit: Stations 3 and 10 are on rest in this circuit.

Figure 10.5 Designing a circuit.

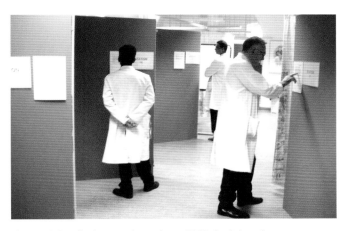

Figure 10.6 A final year undergraduate OSCE circuit in action.

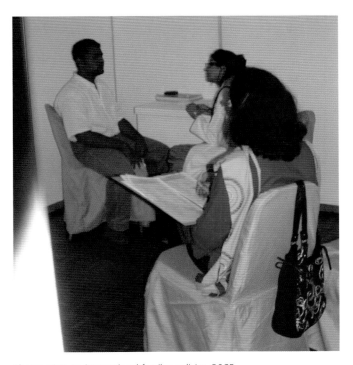

Figure 10.7 An international family medicine OSCE.

'low stakes', fewer longer stations, including examiner feedback, are possible. Provided that the basic principles are followed, the format can be adapted to maximise educational value, improve validity and address feasibility (Figure 10.7).

Station content

Station objectives must be clear and transparent to candidates, simulators and examiners. Increasingly, SBAs rely on simulation using role players (SPs), models or simulators (Figure 10.8). Recruiting and standardising patients is difficult. Where feasible, real patients add authenticity and improve validity.

Aim to integrate the constructs being assessed across stations. This improves both validity and reliability. Careful planning can ensure that skills, for example, communication, are assessed widely across contexts. A SP can be 'attached' to models used for intimate examinations to integrate communication into the skill. Communication, data gathering, diagnosis, management and professionalism may be assessed in all 14 stations (Figure 10.9).

A poor candidate is more reliably identified by performance across all stations. Some argue for single 'killer stations', for example, resuscitation, where unacceptable performance means

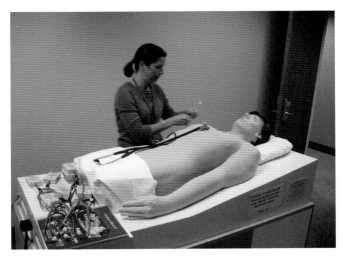

Figure 10.8 Using a simulator.

**LIBRARY
EDUCATION CENTRE
PRINCESS ROYAL HOSPITAL**

Case Reference:	Date of OSCE	Station No:
1 **Consultation Skills**		☐ Excellent
		☐ Competent
		☐ Unsatisfactory
		☐ Poor
2 **Data-gathering Skills**		☐ Excellent
		☐ Competent
		☐ Unsatisfactory
		☐ Poor
3 **Examination and Practical Skills**		☐ Excellent
		☐ Competent
		☐ Unsatisfactory
		☐ Poor
4 **Management and Investigations**		☐ Excellent
		☐ Competent
		☐ Unsatisfactory
		☐ Poor
5 **Professionalism**		☐ Excellent
		☐ Competent
		☐ Unsatisfactory
		☐ Poor
Overall assessment		☐ Excellent
Justification for Pass/Fail Decision		☐ Competent
		☐ Unsatisfactory
Assessor: Date:		☐ Poor

Figure 10.9 An example of a global marking schedule from a postgraduate family medicine skill assessment. It is essential that word descriptors are provided to support the judgements and examiners are trained to use these.

failure overall. This is not advisable. It is unfair to place such weight on one station. Robust standard setting procedures must determine decisions on whether a set number of stations and/or overall mean performance determine pass/fail cut-off scores.

Marking schemes

Scoring against checklists of items is less objective than originally supposed. There is evidence that global ratings, especially by physicians, are equally reliable (Figure 10.9). Neither offers a gold standard for reaching competency judgements. Scoring can be done either by the SP (used in North America) or an examiner.

Training of the marker against the schedule is absolutely essential. They should be familiar with the standard required, understand the criteria and have clear word descriptors (Box 10.2) to define global judgements. Checklists may be more appropriate for undergraduate skills. With developing expertise, global judgements across the constructs being assessed are more appropriate.

> **Box 10.2 Example word descriptor of overall global 'competency' in a patient-centred consultation**
>
> 'Satisfactorily succeeds in demonstrating a caring, patient-centred, holistic approach in an ethical and professional manner, gathering relevant information, performing an appropriate clinical examination and providing largely evidence-based shared management. Is safe for unsupervised practice'.

Evaluation

Figure 10.10 summarises the steps required to deliver a SBA. Evaluating the process is essential. Feedback from candidates is invariably valuable. Examiners and SPs comment constructively on stations. A debrief to review psychometrics, validity and standard setting is essential to ensure a cycle of improvement. Give feedback to all candidates on their performance wherever possible and

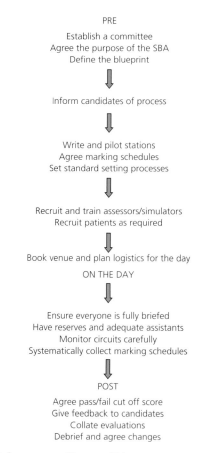

PRE
Establish a committee
Agree the purpose of the SBA
Define the blueprint

Inform candidates of process

Write and pilot stations
Agree marking schedules
Set standard setting processes

Recruit and train assessors/simulators
Recruit patients as required

Book venue and plan logistics for the day
ON THE DAY

Ensure everyone is fully briefed
Have reserves and adequate assistants
Monitor circuits carefully
Systematically collect marking schedules

POST
Agree pass/fail cut off score
Give feedback to candidates
Collate evaluations
Debrief and agree changes

Figure 10.10 Summary – setting up a SBA.

identify poorly performing candidates for further support. These are high-resource tests and educational opportunities must not be overlooked.

Advantages and disadvantages of SBAs

Addressing context specificity is essential to achieve reliability in high-stakes competency skills tests. SBAs remain the best way to ensure the necessary breadth of sampling and standardisation. Traditional long cases and orals logistically cannot do this. The range of examiners involved reduces 'hawk' and 'dove' rater bias.

Validity however is less good. Tasks can become 'atomised'. Integration and authenticity are at risk. SBAs are very resource intensive and yet tend not to be used formatively. WPBA offers opportunities to enhance skills assessment. SBAs, however, remain essential to defensibly assess clinical competency. We need to ensure that the educational opportunities they offer within assessment programmes are not overlooked.

Further reading

Newble D. Techniques for measuring clinical competence: objective structured clinical examinations. *Medical Education* 2004;38:199–203.

References

Downing SM. Reliability: on the reproducibility of assessment data. *Medical Education* 2004;38:1006–1012.

Hodges B. Validity and the OSCE. *Medical Teacher* 2003;25:250–254.

Norcini J. Setting standards on educational tests. *Medical Education* 2003; 37:464–469.

Wass V, Vleuten van der C, Shatzer J, Jones R. Assessment of clinical competence. *Lancet* 2001;357:945–949.

CHAPTER 11

Work-Based Assessment

John Norcini[1] *and Eric Holmboe*[2]

[1] Foundation for Advancement of International Medical Education and Research (FAIMER), Philadelphia, Pennsylvania, USA
[2] American Board of Internal Medicine, Philadelphia, Pennsylvania, USA

OVERVIEW

- Work-based assessments use actual job activities as the grounds for assessment
- The basis for judgements includes patient outcomes, the process of care or the volume of care rendered
- Data can be collected from clinical practice records, administrative databases, diaries and observation
- Portfolios are an aggregation of data from a variety of sources and they require active and ongoing reflection on the part of the doctor

---

In 1990, George Miller proposed a framework for assessing clinical competence (see Chapter 10). At the lowest level of the pyramid is knowledge (knows), followed by competence (knows how), performance (shows how) and action (does). In this framework, Miller distinguished between 'action' and the lower levels. Action focuses on what occurs in practice rather than what happens in an artificial testing situation. Recognising that Miller's framework fails to account for important contextual factors, the Cambridge framework (Figure 11.1) evolved from Miller's pyramid to acknowledge the crucial impact of systems factors (such as interactions with other health-care workers) and individual factors (such as fatigue, illness, etc.).

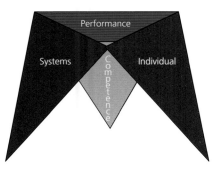

Figure 11.1 Cambridge Model for Assessing Clinical Competence. In this model, the external forces of the health-care system and factors related to the individual doctor (e.g. health, state of mind) play a role in performance.

ABC of Learning and Teaching in Medicine, 2nd edition.
Edited by Peter Cantillon and Diana Wood. © 2010 Blackwell Publishing Ltd.

Work-based methods of assessment target what a doctor does in the context of systems, collecting information about doctors' behaviour in their normal practice. Other common methods of assessment, such as multiple-choice questions, simulation tests and objective structured clinical examinations (OSCEs) target the capacities and capabilities of doctors in controlled settings. Underlying this distinction between performance and action is the sensible but still unproved assumption that assessments of actual practice are a much better reflection of routine performance than assessments done under test conditions.

Methods for work-based assessment

There are many ways to classify work-based assessment methods (Figure 11.2), but in this chapter, they are divided along two dimensions. The first dimension describes the basis for making judgements about the quality of the performance. The second dimension is concerned with how the data are collected. Although the focus of this chapter is on practicing physicians, these same issues apply to the assessment of trainees.

Basis for judgement
Outcomes

In judgements about the outcomes of their patients, the quality of a cardiologist, for example, might be judged by the mortality of his or her patients within 30 days of acute myocardial infarction. Historically, outcomes have been limited to mortality and morbidity, but in

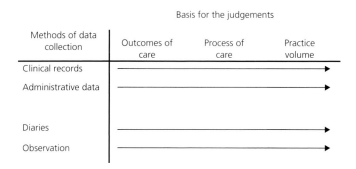

Figure 11.2 Classification scheme for work-based assessment methods.

recent years, the number of clinical end points has been expanded. Patients' satisfaction, functional status, cost-effectiveness and intermediate outcomes – for example, HbA1c and lipid concentrations for diabetic patients – have gained acceptance. Substantial interest has also grown around the problem of diagnostic errors; after all, many of the areas listed above are only useful if based on the right diagnosis. A patient may meet all the quality criteria for asthma, only to be suffering from congestive heart failure.

Patients' outcomes are the best measures of the quality of doctors for the public, the patients and the doctors themselves. For the public, outcomes assessment is a measure of accountability that provides reassurance that the doctor is performing well in practice. For the individual patients, it supplies a basis for deciding which doctor to see. For the doctors, it offers reassurance that their assessment is tailored to their unique practice and based on real-work performance. Despite the fact that an assessment of outcomes is highly desirable, at least five substantial problems remain. These are attribution, complexity, case mix, numbers and detection.

- **Attribution** – for a good judgement to be made about a doctor's performance, the patients' outcomes must be attributable solely to that doctor's actions. This is not realistic when care is delivered within systems and teams. However, recent work has outlined teamwork competencies that are important for physicians and strategies to measure these competencies.
- **Complexity** – patients with the same condition will vary in complexity depending on the severity of their illness, the existence of comorbid conditions and their ability to comply with the doctor's recommendations. Although statistical adjustments may tackle these problems, they are not completely effective. So differences in complexity directly influence outcomes and make it difficult to compare doctors or set standards for their performance.
- **Case mix** – unevenness exists in the case mix of different doctors, again making it difficult to compare performance or to set standards.
- **Numbers** – to estimate a doctor's routine performance well, a sizeable number of patients are needed. This limits outcomes assessment to the most frequently occurring conditions. However, composite measures within and between conditions show substantial promise to address some of the challenges with limited numbers of patients in specific conditions (e.g. diabetes, hypertension, etc.) and improve reliability.
- **Detection** – with regard to diagnostic errors, monitoring systems have to be in place to accurately detect and categorise the error.

Process of care

In judgements about the process of care that doctors provide, a general practitioner, for example, might be assessed on the basis of how many of his or her patients aged over 50 have been screened for colorectal cancer. General process measures include screening, preventive services, diagnosis, management, prescribing, education of patients and counselling. In addition, condition-specific processes might also serve as the basis for making judgements about doctors – for example, whether diabetic patients have their HbA1c monitored regularly and receive routine foot examinations.

Measures of process of care have substantial advantages over outcomes. Firstly, the process of care is more directly in the control of the doctor, so problems of attribution are greatly reduced. Secondly, the measures are less influenced by the complexity of patients' problems – for example, doctors continue to monitor HbA1c regardless of the severity of the diabetes. Thirdly, some of the process measures, such as immunisation, should be offered to all patients of a particular type, reducing the problems of case mix.

The major disadvantage of process measures is that simply doing the right thing does not ensure the best outcomes for patients. While some process measures possess stronger causal links with outcomes, such as immunizations, others such as measuring a haemoglobin A1c do not. That a physician regularly monitors HbA1c, for example, does not guarantee that he or she will make the necessary changes in management. Furthermore, although process measures are less susceptible to the difficulties of attribution, complexity and case mix, these factors still have an adverse influence.

Volume

A third way of assessing the work performance of physicians is by making judgements about the number of times that they have engaged in a particular activity. For example, one measure of quality for a surgeon might be the number of times he or she performed a certain procedure. The premise for this type of assessment is the large body of research indicating that quality of care is associated with higher volume.

Compared to outcomes and process, work-based assessment relying on volume has advantages since problems of attribution are reduced significantly, complexity is eliminated and case mix is not relevant. However, an assessment based on volume alone offers no assurance that the activity was conducted properly.

Method of data collection
Clinical practice records

One of the best sources of information about outcomes, process and volume is the clinical practice record. The external audit of these records is a valid and credible source of data. However, abstracting them is expensive, time-consuming and made cumbersome by the fact that they are often incomplete or illegible. Although it is several years away, widespread adoption of the electronic medical record may be the ultimate solution. Meanwhile, some groups rely on doctors to abstract their own records and submit them for evaluation. Coupled with an external audit of a sample of the participating physicians, this is a credible and feasible alternative.

Administrative databases

Large computerised databases are often developed as part of the process of administering and reimbursing for health care. Data from these sources are accessible, inexpensive and widely available. They can be used in the evaluation of some aspects of practice performance such as cost-effectiveness and medical errors. However, the lack of clinical information and the fact that the data are often collected for billing purposes make them unsuitable as the only source of information.

Diaries

Doctors, especially trainees, often use diaries or logs to keep a record of the procedures they perform. Depending on its purpose, an entry can be accompanied by a description of the physician's role, the name of an observer, an indication of whether it was done properly and a list of complications. This is a reasonable way to collect volume data and an acceptable alternative to clinical practice record abstraction until progress is made with the electronic medical record.

Observation

Data can be collected in many ways through practice observation, but to be consistent with Miller's definition of work-based assessment, the observations need to be routine or covert to avoid an artificial test situation. They can be made in any number of ways and by any number of different observers. The most common forms of observation-based assessment are ratings by supervisors, peers (Table 11.1) and patients (Box 11.1), but nurses and other allied health professionals may also be queried about a doctor's performance. A multi-source feedback (MSF) instrument is simply ratings from some combination of these groups (Lockyer). Other examples of observation include visits by standardised patients (lay people trained to present patient problems realistically) to doctors in their surgeries and audiotapes or videotapes of consultations such as those used by the General Medical Council.

Box 11.1 **An example of a patient rating form**

Below are the types of questions contained in the patient's rating form developed by the American Board of Internal Medicine. Given to 25 patients, it provides a reliable estimate of a doctor's communication skills. The ratings are gathered on a five-point scale (poor to excellent) and they have relationships with validity measures. However, it is important to balance the patients with respect to the age, gender and health status.

Questions:

Tells you everything
Greets you warmly
Treats you like you are on the same level
Let's you tell your story
Shows interest in you as a person
Warns you what is coming during the physical exam
Discusses options
Explains what you need to know
Uses words you can understand

From Webster GD. *Final Report of the Patient Satisfaction Questionnaire Study*. American Board of Internal Medicine, 1989.

Portfolios

Doctors typically collect from various sources the practice data they consider pertinent to their evaluation. A doctor's portfolio might contain data on outcomes, process or volume, collected through clinical record audit, diaries or assessments by patients

---

Table 11.1   An example of a peer evaluation rating form.

Below are the aspects of competence assessed using the peer rating form developed by Ramsey and colleagues. Given to 10 peers, it provides reliable estimates of two overall dimensions of performance: cognitive/clinical skills and professionalism. Ramsey's work indicated that the results are not biased by the method of selecting the peers and they are associated with other measures such as certification status and test scores.

Cognitive/clinical skills
Medical knowledge
Ambulatory care skills
Management of complex problems
Management of hospitalised patients
Problem-solving
Overall clinical competence

Professionalism
Respect
Integrity
Psychosocial aspects of illness
Compassion
Responsibility

From Ramsey PG, Wenrich M, Carline JD, Inui TS, Larson EB, Logerto JP. Use of peer ratings to evaluate physician performance. *JAMA* 1993;269: 1655–1660.

---

and peers (Figure 11.3). It is important to specify what to include in portfolios as doctors will naturally present their best work, and the evaluation of it will not be useful for continuing quality improvement or quality assurance. In addition, if there is a desire to compare doctors or to provide them with feedback about their relative performance, then all portfolios must contain the same data collected in a similar manner. Otherwise, there is no basis for legitimate comparison or benchmarking. Portfolios may be best suited for formative assessment (e.g. feedback) to drive practice-based improvements. Finally, to be effective, portfolios require active and ongoing reflection on the part of the doctor.

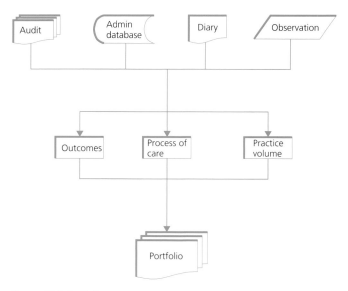

Figure 11.3 Portfolios.

Summary

This chapter defined work-based assessments as occurring in the context of actual job activities. The basis for judgements includes patient outcomes, the process of care or the volume of care rendered. Data can be collected from clinical practice records, administrative databases, diaries and observation. Portfolios are an aggregation of data from a variety of sources and they require active and ongoing reflection on the part of the doctor.

Further reading

Baker DP, Salas E, King H, Battles J, Barach P. The role of teamwork in the professional education of physicians: current status and assessment recommendations. *Joint Commission Journal on Quality and Patient's Safety*. 2005;31:185–202.

Kaplan SH, Griffith JL, Price LL, Pawlson LG, Greenfield S. Improving the reliability of physician performance assessment. Identifying the 'physician effect' on quality and creating composite measures. *Medical Care* 2009;47: 378–387.

Lockyer JM, Clyman SG. Multisource feedback (360-degree evaluation). In Holmboe ES, Hawkins RE, eds. *Practical Guide to the Evaluation of Clinical Competence*. Philadelphia: Mosby-Elsevier, 2008.

McKinley RK, Fraser RC, Baker R. Model for directly assessing and improving competence and performance in revalidation of clinicians. *BMJ* 2001; 322:712.

Rethans JJ, Norcini JJ, Baron-Maldonado M, *et al*. The relationship between competence and performance: implications for assessing practice performance. *Medical Education* 2002;36:901–909.

CHAPTER 12

Direct Observation Tools for Workplace-Based Assessment

Peter Cantillon[1] and Diana Wood[2]

[1]National University of Ireland, Galway, Ireland
[2]University of Cambridge, Cambridge, UK

OVERVIEW

- Assessment tools designed to facilitate the direct observation of learners' performance in the workplace are now widely used in both undergraduate and postgraduate medical education

- Direct observation tools represent a compromise between tests of competence and performance and offer a practical means of evaluating 'on-the-job' performance

- Most of the direct observation tools available assess single encounters and thus require multiple observations by different assessors

- Multi-source feedback methods described in this chapter represent an alternative to single encounter assessments and provide a means of assessing routine practice

Introduction

The assessment of doctors' performance in practice remains a major challenge. While tests of competence assess a doctor's ability to perform a task on a single occasion, measurement of performance in daily clinical practice is more difficult. Assessment of many different aspects of work may be desirable such as decision-making, teamwork and professionalism, but these are not amenable to traditional methods of assessment. In this chapter, we will describe assessment tools designed to facilitate the direct observation of doctors performing functions in the workplace. These approaches differ from those described in Chapter 11 in that they measure doctor's performance under observation. Deliberate observation of a trainee or student using a rating tool represents an artificial intervention and cannot be regarded as a measure of how a doctor might act when unobserved. However, although representing a compromise between tests of competence and performance, these tests have been widely adopted as a practical means of evaluating 'on-the-job' performance.

Direct observation

Direct observation of medical trainees working with patients by clinical supervisors is an essential feature of teaching and assessing

ABC of Learning and Teaching in Medicine, 2nd edition.
Edited by Peter Cantillon and Diana Wood. © 2010 Blackwell Publishing Ltd.

clinical and communication skills. The assessment tools described in this chapter represent the products of a deliberate effort in recent years to design measures of the quality of observed learner behaviour.

Direct observation formats are usually designed to assess single encounters, for example, the mini-clinical evaluation exercise (mini-CEX), the direct observation of procedural skills (DOPS) and the chart stimulated recall tool or case-based discussion (CSR, CBD). An alternative approach is to record the observation of performance over time (i.e. what the doctor does day to day and over a period of time). A good example is the multi-source feedback (MSF) approach, such as the mini-PAT. One of the major advantages of all these methods is that they allow for immediate formative feedback.

Single encounter tools
The mini-CEX

The mini-CEX is an observation tool that facilitates the assessment of skills that are essential for good clinical care and the provision of immediate feedback. In a mini-CEX assessment, the tutor observes the learner's interaction with a patient in a clinical setting. Typically, the student or trainee carries out a focused clinical activity (taking a clinical history, examining a system, etc.) and provides a summary. Using a global rating sheet the teacher scores the performance and gives feedback. Mini-CEX encounters should take between 10 and 15 minutes duration with 5 minutes for feedback. Typically during a period of 1 year a trainee would be assessed on several occasions by different assessors using the mini-CEX tool (Figure 12.1). By involving different assessors the mini-CEX assessment reduces the bias associated with the single observer. The assessment of multiple samples of the learner's performance in different domains addresses the case specificity of a single observation. The mini-CEX is used for looking at aspects of medical interviewing, physical examination, professionalism, clinical judgement, counselling, communication skills, organisation and efficiency, as well as overall clinical competence. It is intended to identify students or trainees whose performance is unsatisfactory as well as to provide competent students with appropriate formative feedback. It is not intended for use in high-stakes assessment or for comparison between trainees. The number of observations necessary to get a reliable picture of a trainee's performance varies between four and eight. The poorer a student or trainee, the more observations are

RCP MINI CLINICAL EVALUATION EXERCISE

Assessor's GMC Number   **SpR's GMC Number**

Date (DD/MM/YY)

☐☐ / ☐☐ / ☐☐

Year of SpR training

○ 1 ○ 2 ○ 3 ○ 4 ○ 5 ○ 6

Patient problem/Diagnosis:

Case Setting   ○ Out-patient   ○ In-patient   ○ A&E   Is the patient: ○ New   ○ Follow-up?
Case Complexity: ○ Low   ○ Moderate   ○ High
Focus of mini-CEX: (more than one may be selected)   ○ Data Gathering   ○ Diagnosis   ○ Management   ○ Counselling
What type of consultation was this?   ○ Good news   ○ Bad news   ○ Neither

Please mark one of the circle for each component of the exercise on a scale of 1 (extremely poor) to 9 (extremely good). A score of 1–3 is considered unsatisfactory, 4–6 satisfactory and 7–9 is considered above that expected, for a trainee at the same stage of training and level of experience. Please note that your scoring should reflect the performance of the SpR against that which you would reasonably expect at their stage of training and level of experience. You must justify each score of 1–3 with at least one explanation/example in the comments box, failure to do so will invalidate the assessment. Please feel free to add any other relevant opinions about this doctor's strengths and weaknesses.

1. Medical Interviewing Skills
○ Not observed or applicable ○ 1   ○ 2   ○ 3   ○ 4   ○ 5   ○ 6   ○ 7   ○ 8   ○ 9
                              UNSATISFACTORY   SATISFACTORY   ABOVE EXPECTED

2. Physical Examination Skills
○ Not observed or applicable ○ 1   ○ 2   ○ 3   ○ 4   ○ 5   ○ 6   ○ 7   ○ 8   ○ 9

3. Consideration For Patient/Professionalism
○ Not observed or applicable ○ 1   ○ 2   ○ 3   ○ 4   ○ 5   ○ 6   ○ 7   ○ 8   ○ 9

4. Clinical Judgement
○ Not observed or applicable ○ 1   ○ 2   ○ 3   ○ 4   ○ 5   ○ 6   ○ 7   ○ 8   ○ 9

5. Counselling and Communication skills
○ Not observed or applicable ○ 1   ○ 2   ○ 3   ○ 4   ○ 5   ○ 6   ○ 7   ○ 8   ○ 9

6. Organisation/Efficiency
○ Not observed or applicable ○ 1   ○ 2   ○ 3   ○ 4   ○ 5   ○ 6   ○ 7   ○ 8   ○ 9

7. OVERALL CLINICAL COMPETENCE
                              ○ 1   ○ 2   ○ 3   ○ 4   ○ 5   ○ 6   ○ 7   ○ 8   ○ 9

Assessor's comments on trainee's performance on this occasion (BLOCK CAPITALS PLEASE)

Trainee's comments on their performance on this occasion (BLOCK CAPITALS PLEASE)

Trainee's signature

Assessor's signature

Figure 12.1 Example of mini-CEX assessment: mini-CEX evaluation form. Royal College of Physicians of London: www.rcplondon.ac.uk/education.

Direct Observation of Procedural Skills (DOPS) – Anaesthesia

Please complete the questions using a cross (x). Please use black ink and CAPITAL LETTERS.

Trainee's surname:

Trainee's forename(s):

GMC number: **GMC NUMBER MUST BE COMPLETED**

Clinical setting: Theatre ☐ ICU ☐ A&E ☐ Delivery suite ☐ Pain clinic ☐ Other ☐

Procedure:

Case category: Elective ☐ Scheduled ☐ Urgent ☐ Emergency ☐ Other ☐ ASA Class: 1 2 3 4 5

Assessor's position: Consultant ☐ SASG ☐ SpR ☐ Nurse ☐ Other ☐

Number of times previous DOPS observed by assessor with **any** trainee: 0 ☐ 1 ☐ 2–5 ☐ 5–9 ☐ >9 ☐

Number of times procedure performed byt rainee: 0 ☐ 1–4 ☐ 5–9 ☐ >10 ☐

Please grade the following areas using the scale below:	Below expectations		Borderline	Meets expectations	Above expectations		U/C*
	1	2	3	4	5	6	
1	Demonstrates understanding of indications, relevant anatomy, technique of procedure						
2	Obtains informed consent						
3	Demonstrates appropriate pre-procedure preparation						
4	Demonstrates situation awareness						
5	Aseptic technique						
6	Technical ability						
7	Seeks help where appropriate						
8	Post procedure management						
9	Communication skills						
10	Consideration for patient						
11	Overall performance						

*U/C Please mark this if you have not observed the behaviour and therefore feel unable to comment.

Please use this space to record areas of strength or any suggestions for development.

Not at all   Highly

Trainee satisfaction with DOPS: 1 ☐ 2 ☐ 3 ☐ 4 ☐ 5 ☐ 6 ☐ 7 ☐ 8 ☐ 9 ☐ 10 ☐

Assessor satisfaction with DOPS: 1 ☐ 2 ☐ 3 ☐ 4 ☐ 5 ☐ 6 ☐ 7 ☐ 8 ☐ 9 ☐ 10 ☐

What training have you had in the use of this assessment tool? Face-to-face ☐ Have read guidelines ☐ Web/CDROM ☐

Assessor's signature:... Date:.................................

Time taken for observation (in minutes): ☐☐ Time taken for feedback (in minutes): ☐☐

Assessor's name:

Assessor's GMC number: *Acknowledgement: Adapted with permission from the American Board of Internal Medicine.*

PLEASE NOTE: failure to return all completed forms to your administrator is a probity issue.

Figure 12.2 Example of DOPS assessment: DOPS evaluation form. Royal College of Anaesthetists: http://www.rcoa.ac.uk/docs/DOPS.pdf.

Direct Observation of Procedural Skills (DOPS)

DOPS assessment takes the form of the trainee performing a specific practical procedure that is directly observed and scored by a consultant observer in each of the eleven domains, using the standard form.

Performing a DOPS assessment will slow down the procedure but the principal burden is providing an assessor at the time that a skilled trainee will be performing the practical task.

Being a practical specialty there are numerous examples of procedures that require assessment as detailed in each unit of training. The assessment of each procedure should focus on the whole event, not simply, for example, the successful insertion of cannula, the location of epidural space or central venous access such that, in the assessors' judgment the trainee is competent to perform the individual procedure without direct supervision.

Feedback and discussion at the end of the session is mandatory.

Figure 12.2 *continued.*

necessary. For example, in the United Kingdom, the Foundation Programme recommends that each trainee should have between four and six mini-CEX evaluations in any year. The mini-CEX has been extensively adapted since its original introduction in 1995 to suit the nature of different clinical specialties and different levels of expected trainee competence.

The mini-CEX has been widely adopted as it is relatively quick to do, provides excellent observation data for feedback and has been validated in numerous settings. However, the challenges of running a clinical service frequently take precedence and it can be difficult to find the time to do such focused observations. Differences in the degree of challenge between different cases lead to variance in scores achieved.

Direct Observation of Procedural Skills

The DOPS tool was designed by the Royal College of Physicians (Figure 12.2) as an adaptation of the mini-CEX to specifically assess performance of practical clinical procedures. Just as in the case of the mini-CEX, the trainee usually selects a procedure from an approved list and agrees on a time and place for a DOPS assessment by a supervisor. The scoring is similar to that of the mini-CEX and is based on a global rating scale. As with the mini-CEX, the recording sheet encourages the assessor to record the setting, the focus, the complexity of the case, the time of the consultation and the feedback given. Typically, a DOPS assessment will review the indications for the procedure, how consent was obtained, whether appropriate analgesia (if necessary) was used, technical ability, professionalism, clinical judgement and awareness of complications. Trainees are usually assessed six or more times a year looking at a range of procedures and employing different observers.

There are a large number of procedures that can be assessed by DOPS across many specialties. Reported examples include skin biopsy, autopsy procedures, histology procedures, handling and reporting of frozen sections, operative skills and insertion of central lines. The advantage of the DOPS assessment is that it allows one to directly assess clinical procedures and to provide immediate structured feedback. DOPS is now being used commonly in specialties that involve routine procedural activities.

Chart stimulated recall (case-based discussion)

The Chart Stimulated Recall (CSR) assessment was developed in the United States in the context of emergency medicine. In the United Kingdom, this assessment is called Case-based Discussion (CBD). In CSR/CBD the assessor is interested in the quality of the trainee's diagnostic reasoning, his/her rationale for choosing certain actions and their awareness of differential diagnosis. In a typical CSR/CBD assessment (Figure 12.3), the trainee selects several cases for discussion and the assessor picks one for review. The assessor asks the trainee to describe the case and asks clarifying questions. Once the salient details of the case have been shared, the assessor focuses on the trainee's thinking and decision-making in relation to selected aspects of the case such as investigative or therapeutic strategy. CSR/CBD is designed to stimulate discussion about a case so that the assessor can get a sense of the trainee's knowledge, reasoning and awareness of ethical issues. It is of particular value in clinical specialties where understanding of laboratory techniques and interpretation of results is crucial such as endocrinology, clinical biochemistry and radiology. CSR/CBD is another single-encounter observation method and as such multiple measures need to be taken to reduce case specificity. Thus it is usual to arrange four to six encounters of CSR/CBD during any particular year carried out by different assessors. CSR/CBD has been shown to be good at detecting poorly performing doctors and correlates well with other forms of cognitive assessment. As with the DOPS and mini-CEX assessments, lack of time to carry out observations and inconsistency in the use of the instrument can undermine its effectiveness.

Multiple source feedback

It is much harder to measure routine practice compared with assessing single encounters. Most single-encounter measures, such as those described above, are indirect, that is, they look at the products of routine practice rather than the practice itself. One method that looks at practice more directly albeit through the eyes of peers is multiple source feedback (MSF). MSF tools represent a way in which the perspectives of colleagues and patients can be collected and collated in a systematic manner so that they can be used to both assess performance and at the same time provide a source of feedback for doctors in training.

A commonly used MSF tool in the United Kingdom is the mini-PAT (mini-Peer Assessment Technique), a shortened version of the Sheffield Peer Review Assessment Tool (SPRAT) (Figure 12.4). In a typical mini-PAT assessment, the trainee selects eight assessors representing a mix of senior supervisors, trainee colleagues, nursing colleagues, clinic staff and so on. Each assessor

LIBRARY
EDUCATION CENTRE
PRINCESS ROYAL HOSPITAL

The Royal College of Pathologists
Pathology: the science behind the cure

WORKPLACE-BASED ASSESSMENT FORM

CHEMICAL PATHOLOGY

Case-based discussion (CbD)

Trainee's name:		GMC N°:		Stage of training: A B C D

Assessor's name:		Please circle one	Consultant SAS Senior BMS Clinical scientist Trainee Other

Brief outline of procedure, indicating focus for assessment (refer to topics in curriculum). Tick category of case or write in space below.

- [ ] Biological variation pregnancy/childhood
- [ ] Liver Gastroenterology
- [ ] Lipids CVS
- [ ] Diabetes Endocrinology
- [ ] Nutrition
- [ ] Calcium/Bone Magnesium
- [ ] Water/electrolytes Urogenital
- [ ] Gas transport [H+] metabolism
- [ ] Proteins Enzymology
- [ ] IMD
- [ ] Genetics Molecular Biology
- [ ] Please specify:

Complexity of procedure: [ ] Low [ ] Average [ ] High

Please ensure this patient is not identifiable

Please grade the following areas using the scale provided. This should relate to the standard expected for the end of the appropriate stage of training:

		Below expectations	Borderline	Meets expectations	Above expectations		Unable to comment
		1	2	3	4	5	6	
1	Understanding of theory of case							
2	Clinical assessment of case							
3	Additional investigations (e.g. appropriateness, cost effectiveness)							
4	Consideration of laboratory issues							
5	Action and follow-up							
6	Advice to clinical users							
7	Overall clinical judgement							
8	Overall professionalism							

PLEASE COMMENT TO SUPPORT YOUR SCORING:

SUGGESTED DEVELOPMENTAL WORK:
(particularly areas scoring 1–3)

Outcome:	Satisfactory Unsatisfactory (Please circle as appropriate)	Date of assessment:		Time taken for assessment:	
Signature of assessor:		Signature of trainee:		Time taken for feedback:	

Figure 12.3 Example of CSR/CBD assessment: CBD evaluation form. Royal College of Pathologists: http://www.rcpath.org/resources/pdf/Chemical_pathology_CbD_form.pdf.

ISCP INTERCOLLEGIATE SURGICAL CURRICULUM PROGRAMME

Self Mini-PAT (Peer Assessment Tool)

Please complete the questions using a cross: ☒ Please use black ink and CAPITAL LETTERS

Your forename:

Your surname:

Your GMC number:　　　　　Hospital:

Trainee level:　ST1 ☐　ST2 ☐　ST3 ☐　ST4 ☐　ST5 ☐　ST6 ☐　ST7 ☐　ST 8 ☐　Other ＿＿＿

Specialty:　☐　　☐　　☐　　☐　　☐　　☐　　☐　　☐　　☐
　　　　　Cardio　General　Neuro　O&M　Otol　Paed　Plast　T&O　Urology

How do you rate yourself in your:	Standard: The assessment should be judged against the standard expected at completion of this level of training. Levels of training are defined in the syllabus						
	Below expectations		Borderline	Meets expectations	Above expectations		U/C[1]
	1	2	3	4	5	6	
Good Clinical Care							
1. Ability to diagnose patient problems							
2. Ability to formulate appropriate management plans							
3. Awareness of own limitations							
4. Ability to respond to psychosocial aspects of illness							
5. Appropriate utilisation of resources e.g. ordering investigations							
Maintaining good medical practice							
6. Ability to manage time effectively/ prioritise							
7. Technical skills (appropriate to current practice)							
Teaching and Training, Appraising and Assessing							
8. Willingness and effectiveness when teaching/training colleagues							
Relationship with Patients							
9. Communication with patients							
10. Communication with carers and/or family							
11. Respect for patients and their right to confidentiality							
Working with colleagues							
12. Verbal communication with colleagues							
13. Written communication with colleagues							
14. Ability to recognise and value the contribution of others							
15. Accessibility/Reliability							
Overall							
16. Overall, how do you compare yourself to a doctor ready to complete this level of training?							

[1] U/C Please mark this if you feel unable to comment.

Acknowledgements: Mini-PAT is derived from SPRAT (Sheffield Peer Review Assessment Tool)

PTO:

Figure 12.4 Example of mini-PAT assessment: mini-PAT evaluation form. Royal College of Surgeons: https://www.iscp.ac.uk/static/public/minipat_self_form.pdf.

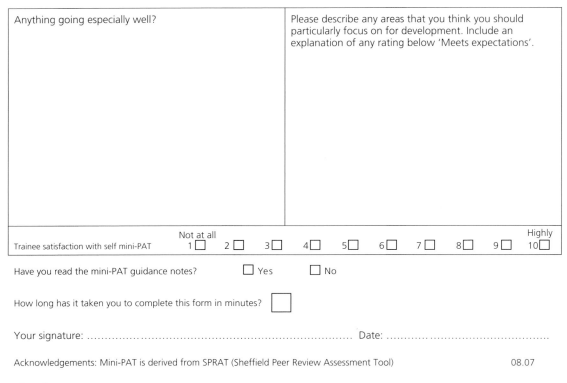

Figure 12.4 *continued.*

is sent a mini-PAT questionnaire to complete. The trainee also self-assesses using the mini-PAT questionnaire. The questionnaire requires each assessor to rate various aspects of the trainee's work such as relationships with patients and interaction with colleagues. The questionnaire data from the peer assessors are amalgamated and, when presented to the trainee, are offered in a manner that allows the trainee to see his/her self-rating compared with the mean ratings of the peer assessors. Trainees can also compare their ratings to national mean ratings in the United Kingdom. The results are reviewed by the educational supervisor with the trainee and together they agree on what is working well and what aspects of clinical, professional or team performance need more work. In the United Kingdom, this process is usually repeated twice a year for the duration of the trainee's training programme.

Training assessors

Assessors are the major source of variance in performance-based assessment. There is good evidence to show that with adequate training variance between assessors is reduced and that assessors gain both reliability and confidence in their use of these tools. Assessors need to be aware of what to look for with different clinical presentations and with different levels of trainees and need to understand the dimensions of performance that are being measured and how these are reflected in the tool itself. They should be given the opportunity to practise direct observation tools using

live or videotaped examples of performance. Assessors should be then encouraged to compare their judgements with standardised marking schedules or with colleagues so that they can begin to calibrate themselves and improve their accuracy and discrimination.

Maximum benefit from workplace-based assessments is gained when they are accompanied by skilled and expert feedback. Assessors should be trained to give effective formative feedback.

Problems with direct observation methods

While direct observation of practice in the work place remains one of the best means available for assessing integrated skills in the context of patient care, the fact that the trainee and supervisor have to interrupt their clinical practice in order to carry out an assessment means that neither is behaving normally and that the time required represents a significant feasibility challenge. In direct observation methods, the relationship between the trainee and the assessor may be a source of positive or negative bias, hence the need for multiple assessors. When used for progression requirements, direct observation tools may be problematic given the natural tendency to avoid negative evaluations. Assessor training and the use of external examiners may help to alleviate this problem, but it is arguable that the direct observation tools should not be used in high-stakes assessments.

Direct observations of single encounters should not represent the only form of assessment in the workplace. In the case of poorly performing trainee a direct observation method may identify a problem that needs to be further assessed with another tool such as a cognitive test of knowledge. Moreover, differences in the relative difficulty of cases used in assessing a group of equivalently experienced trainees can also lead to errors of measurement. This problem can be partially addressed through careful selection of cases and attention to the level of difficulty for each trainee. It is also true that assessors themselves may rate cases as more or less complex, depending on their level of expertise with such cases in their own practice. Thus it is essential with all of these measures to use multiple observations as a single observation is a poor predictor of a doctor's performance in other settings with other cases.

Conclusion

Direct observation methods are a valuable, albeit theoretically flawed, addition to the process of assessment of a student or doctor's performance in practice. Appropriately used in a formative manner, they can give useful information about progression through an educational programme and highlight areas for further training.

Further reading

Archer J. Assessment and appraisal. In Cooper N, Forrest K, eds. *Essential Guide to Educational Supervision in Postgraduate Medical Education.* Oxford: BMJ Books, Wiley Blackwell, 2009.

Archer JC, Norcini J, Davies HA. Peer review of paediatricians in training using SPRAT. *BMJ* 2005;330:1251–1253.

Norcini J. Workplace-based assessment in clinical training. In Swanwick T, ed. *Understanding Medical Education.* Edinburgh: ASME, 2007.

Norcini J, Burch V. Workplace-based assessment as an educational tool. *Medical Teacher* 2007;29:855–871.

Wood DF. Formative assessment. In Swanwick T, ed. *Understanding Medical Education.* Edinburgh: ASME, 2007.

CHAPTER 13

Learning Environment

Jill Thistlethwaite

University of Warwick, Coventry, UK

OVERVIEW

- A supportive environment promotes active and deep learning
- Learning needs to be transferred from the classroom to clinical settings
- Educators have less control over clinical environments, which are unpredictable
- Learners need roles within their environments and their tasks should become more complex as they become more senior
- Virtual learning environments are used frequently to complement learning

The skills and knowledge of individual teachers are only some of the factors that influence how, why and what learners learn. Learners do best when they are immersed in an environment that supports and promotes active and deep learning. This environment includes not only the physical space or setting but also the people within it. It is a place where learners and teachers interact and socialise and also where education involves the wider community, particularly in those settings outside the academic walls. Everyone should feel as comfortable as possible within the environment: learners, educators, health professionals, patients, staff and visitors. In health professional education, the learning environment includes the settings listed in Box 13.1.

Box 13.1 **Different learning environments**

- Classroom
- Laboratory (including clinical skills)
- Lecture theatre
- Library
- Patient's home
- Ward
- Outpatient department
- Emergency department
- Community setting including general practice
- Virtual learning environment (VLE)
- Learner's home

ABC of Learning and Teaching in Medicine, 2nd edition.
Edited by Peter Cantillon and Diana Wood. © 2010 Blackwell Publishing Ltd.

Transfer of learning

Health professional students, including medical students, need to be flexible to the demands of the environments through which they rotate. A key concept is the transfer of learning from one setting to another: from the classroom to the ward, from the lecture theatre to the surgical theatre, from the clinical skills laboratory to a patient's home. This transfer is helped by the move in modern medical education to case- and problem-based learning away from didactic lectures, and an emphasis on reasoning rather than memorising facts. However, sometimes previous learning inhibits or interferes with education in a new setting or context. A student, who has received less than glowing feedback while practising communication skills with simulated patients, may feel awkward and reticent interacting with patients who are ill.

For qualified health professionals, the learning environment is often contiguous with the workplace. Learning takes place in the clinical setting if time is available for reflection and learning from experience, including from critical incidents using tools such as clinical event analysis. Boud and Walker (1990) developed a conceptual model of learning from experience, which includes what they termed the *learning milieu* where experience facilitates action through reflection (Figure 13.1).

Case history 1 – Confidentiality in the classroom

A student group is discussing self-care and their personal experiences of ill health and consulting with doctors. One student volunteers information about an eating disorder she had while at secondary school. The group facilitator is also a clinician at one of the teaching hospitals. A few weeks later some of the students attend a lunchtime lecture at the hospital for clinicians given by the facilitator. The doctor illustrates the topic with reference to a case of anorexia that the student recognises as her own.

Learning point: Ground rules for group work must include discussion about confidentiality.

Essential components of the learning environment

Medical educators have more control over the medical school environment than they do over other settings. Universities provide

LIBRARY
EDUCATION CENTRE
PRINCESS ROYAL HOSPITAL

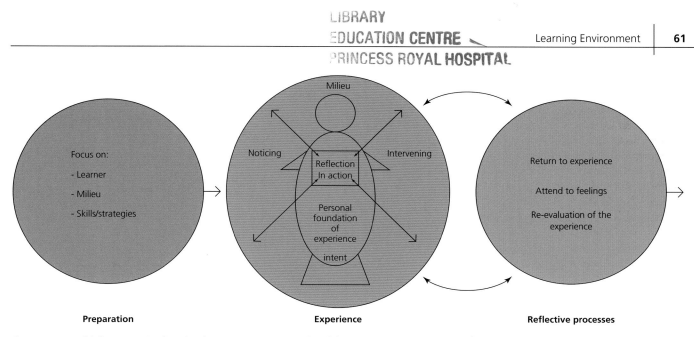

Figure 13.1 Model for promoting learning from experience. Reproduced from Boud D, Walker D. Making the most of experience. *Studies in Continuing Education* 1990;12:61–80. With permission from Taylor and Francis Ltd. www.informaworld.com.

learners with access to resources for facilitating learning such as a library, the Internet and discussion rooms (both real and virtual). Learning tools are usually up to date and computers up to speed. However, once learners venture outside the higher education institution, and later in their careers as doctors, these resources may not be as available. Features of an optimal learning environment include physical and social factors (Box 13.2). In addition, the learning milieu also implies attention to features of good educational delivery such as organisation, clear learning goals and outcomes, flexible delivery and timely feedback. Adult learners should also have some choice of what is learnt and how it is learnt.

Box 13.2 **Features of optimum learning environments (physical, social and virtual)**

- Commitment of all those within the setting to high-quality education
- Appropriate temperature
- Airy
- Adequate space (can move without disturbing others)
- Natural light
- Minimal outside noise
- Comfortable to write in
- Free from hazards
- Stimulating
- Availability of appropriate refreshment
- Adaptability for disabled participants
- Non-threatening – what is said in the setting remains in the setting
- Opportunity for social as well as educational interaction
- Supportive staff
- Appropriate workload
- Functionality
- Easy to access
- Accessibility from different locations
- Different levels of accessibility
- Confidential material – password protected

Educators within the learning environment should be aware of their learners' prior experiences.

Educators rarely have the luxury of designing a new building, which allows a seamless movement between formal and informal teaching and socialisation. While we cannot alter the shape, we can make the entrance more welcoming with good signage and cheerful receptionists. This is particularly important for the patients and service users involved in activities as educators or learners.

Room layout and facilities are important factors in the delivery of education. Clear instructions to the relevant administrators are essential before delivering a session, particularly if there is a visiting educator. The room should be of the right size for the number of people expected – too small and learners are cramped and feel undervalued; too large and all participants, including the educator, feel uncomfortable. Do the chairs need to be in a circle? Are tables required, a flip chart or white board? Computer facilities should be checked for compatibility with prepared presentations. For learning sessions involving technology, there should be a technician available if things go wrong – keeping the process running smoothly is so important to avoid tutor burnout and student apathy.

Clinical environments

When considering the delivery of health professional education, and the clinical settings in which it takes place, it is obvious that the environment is often less than satisfactory. Educators have less control over clinical spaces, which often have suboptimal features. Wards are overheated (or over-air-conditioned in the tropics), patients and staff may overhear conversations, students stand for long periods of time during ward rounds and bedside teaching or may be inactive waiting 'for something to happen'. Clinical environments are often noisy and potentially hazardous. Community settings can be more ambient, but confidentiality may still be a problem. Clinical environments should promote situated learning, that is, learning embedded in the social and physical settings in which it will be used.

Learning is promoted if students feel part of the clinical team and have real work to do, within the limits of their competence. Learning in clinical environments is still carried out through a form of apprenticeship, a community of practice as defined by Lave and Wenger (1991). In this community, students learn by participation and by contributing to tasks which have meaning, a process called 'legitimate peripheral participation'. They need to feel valued and should not be undermined by negative feedback, particularly in front of others. Bullying and intimidation have no place in modern education. Clinical tutors and staff should intervene if students do not act professionally with peers, patients or colleagues. Everyone in the clinical environment is a role model and should be aware of this.

Learners new to a particular setting need to have an orientation and clear preparatory instructions including how to dress appropriately for the setting. The pervading culture of the environment is important. We often forget that clinical environments are unfamiliar to many students – they may feel unwanted and underfoot. They feel unsure of the hierarchy operating around them; who should they ask about patients, where can they find torches, how can they access patients' records or are they allowed to access results? Is the ward, outpatient department or GP's surgery welcoming? Orientation is important for even such simple points as where to hang a coat, where to find the toilet or where to go to have a cup of tea. During clinical attachments, students may encounter death and dying for the first time, without a chance to discuss their feelings or debrief. They may see patient–professional interactions that upset them; they will almost certainly be exposed to black humour and initially find it unsettling and then, worryingly, join in to fit in (the influence of the hidden curriculum). The process of professional socialisation begins early.

An even more unsettling and new environment with its different culture and dress code is the operating theatre. Here novices may become so anxious about doing the wrong thing that meaningful learning is unlikely. Lyon (2003) suggested that students have to manage their learning across three domains, not only needing to become familiar with the physical environment with attention to sterility but also with new social relations while concentrating on their own tasks and learning outcomes. Though modern operating techniques make it unlikely that a student will have to stand motionless with a retractor for several hours, they may have physical discomfort from trying to observe, straining to listen and even not being able to take notes. The skilful surgeon or nurse educator in this situation will ensure that students are able to participate and reflect on what is happening and make them feel part of the team by suggesting tasks within their capabilities.

Case history 2 – Consideration for patients

Two final year students are attached to the emergency department of a large hospital. A patient is admitted with abdominal pain and the specialist registrar (SpR) asks the students to take a history. The students introduce themselves to the patient who says he does not want to talk to students – where is the doctor? The SpR is annoyed and says that they should have let the man assume they were junior doctors. The students feel uncomfortable but want the SpR to teach them – they are unsure of what to do. Later the SpR asks one of the students to take an arterial blood sample from another patient. She advises that the student asks the patient for consent but not to tell the patient that this is the student's first time of doing this procedure.

Learning points: All staff who interact with learners need to behave professionally. Students should know who they can contact if they feel they are being asked to do anything that makes them feel uncomfortable.

Increasing seniority

As learners become more senior there needs to be a balance between autonomy and supervision. While junior students need a well-structured timetable, clear instructions and targets, in the later years and after qualification, learners use personal development plans to guide their learning and have greater flexibility in what they do.

Of course, learning does not stop at the university; one of the aims of undergraduate education is to equip doctors and health professionals with the skills for lifelong learning. Therefore, the workplace is also an environment in which learning needs to be balanced with service commitment. Teaching may still be formalised, but it is often opportunistic and trainees require time to reflect on their clinical experiences and daily duties. While there may be more kudos from working in a large tertiary teaching hospital, junior doctors often prefer the more manageable smaller district hospital where they know the staff and where they are more likely to be seen as individuals, and can understand the organisation of the workplace.

Workload is a contentious point. Students usually feel they are overworked; tutors think that students have too much free time. Junior medical students may be working to supplement their loans; mature students may have family demands. Junior doctors have to learn to balance service commitment, education and outside life. Professionals undertaking continuing professional development (CPD) usually have full-time jobs and fit in formal learning activities after work when they are tired and mulling over daytime incidents.

Virtual learning environments (VLE)

The definition of a VLE by the Joint Information Systems Committee (JISC) is shown in Box 13.3. This electronic environment supports education through its online tools, discussion rooms, databases and resources and, as with 'real' learning environments, there is an etiquette and optimal ambience associated with it. VLEs do not operate by themselves and need planning, evaluation and support. Content needs to be kept up to date; otherwise, users will move elsewhere. The VLE may contain resources previously available in paper form such as lecture notes, reading lists and recommended articles. It should, however, move beyond being a repository only of paper artefacts and encompass innovative and value-added electronic learning objects.

Box 13.3 JISC definitions of MLE and VLE

The term **Managed Learning Environment (MLE)** is used to include the whole range of information systems and processes of a college (including its VLE if it has one) that contribute directly, or indirectly, to learning and the management of that learning.

The term **Virtual Learning Environment (VLE)** is used to refer to the 'online' interactions of various kinds which take place between learners and tutors. The JISC MLE Steering Group has said that VLE refers to the components in which learners and tutors participate in 'online' interactions of various kinds, including online learning.

Accessed from: http://www.jisc.ac.uk/index.cfm?name=mle_briefings_1

Within health professional education the VLE cannot take the place of authentic experiences and learner–patient interactions but can assist in providing opportunities to learn from and about patients in other settings, to discuss with learners at distant locations and to provide material generated at one institution to be interacted with at another (through lecture streaming, for example). Thus the VLE facilitates the community of practice. VLEs can be expensive; they require technical support and good security. Too much reliance on technology is frustrating when systems crash, and not all learners feel comfortable with them.

Evaluation of the learning environment

The learning environment should be regularly evaluated as part of feedback from learners and educators, plus patients and other clinical staff as appropriate. There are a number of validated tools to help with this, including the Dundee Ready Education Environment Measure (DREEM). This has five subscales (Box 13.4) and has been

Box 13.4 DREEM subscales

- Students' perceptions of learning
- Students' perceptions of teaching
- Students' academic self-perception
- Students' perception of atmosphere
- Students' social self-perception

used widely and internationally. The evaluation needs to be acted upon, and seen to be acted upon, to close the feedback loop. Learners become disillusioned with evaluation forms if they feel they are not being listened to and nothing changes.

Recommendations to enhance learning environments

- Ensure adequate orientation.
- Know what learners have already covered and build on this.
- Do not stand too long round a bedside – it is difficult for the patient and learners.
- Keep sessions short, or have comfort breaks.
- Watch learners' body language for discomfort and disquiet.
- Watch patients' body language for discomfort and disquiet.
- Ensure time for debriefing of learners regularly, particularly after clinical interactions and attachments.
- Be prepared – familiarise yourself with the room and the technology where you will be teaching.
- Ensure the room is arranged the best way for your teaching style/session.
- Ensure that participants know where the exits and toilets are, when there are breaks and refreshments.
- Do not forget about the need to enhance the learning environment for non-academic teachers/facilitators including patient-educators.

Further reading

Joint Information Systems Committee, available at: http://www.jisc.ac.uk/

Roff S, McAleer S, Harden RM *et al*. Development and validation of the Dundee Ready Education Environment Measure. *Medical Teacher* 1997;19: 295–299.

References

Boud D, Walker D. Making the most of experience. *Studies in Continuing Education* 1990;12:61–80.

Lave J, Wenger E. *Situated Learning: Legitimate Peripheral Participation*. Melbourne: Cambridge University Press, 1991.

Lyon P. Making the most of learning in the operating theatre: student strategies and curricular initiatives. *Medical Education* 2003;37:680–688.

CHAPTER 14

Creating Teaching Materials

Jean Ker and Anne Hesketh

University of Dundee, Dundee, UK

OVERVIEW

- Teaching materials include a broad church from paper to simulation exercises
- Use CREATE principles to develop teaching materials
- Use teaching materials to enhance best conditions for learning
- Explore whether resources are already available to avoid duplication
- Plan how to evaluate the educational impact of the teaching materials

Introduction

In this chapter we will outline guidelines to produce effective teaching materials and highlight some of the pitfalls to avoid. All medical teachers should use a system to design instructional materials which create the right conditions for learning.

When we think of teaching materials we usually think of lecture notes and handouts but in today's world, we also need to think of simulation, study guides and Virtual Learning Environments (VLEs). In relation to the purpose and context of teaching materials, we also need to consider how to effectively support the independent learner.

Getting started

Some key questions to answer when you need to develop new teaching materials are as follows:

- Why are teaching materials needed?
- What are the different mediums that can be used to create teaching materials?
- Who should create teaching resources?
- What influences the creation of effective learning materials?

ABC of Learning and Teaching in Medicine, 2nd edition.
Edited by Peter Cantillon and Diana Wood. © 2010 Blackwell Publishing Ltd.

Guiding principles for creating teaching materials

There are six guiding principles that will help you as a teacher answer these questions captured by the acronym CREATE (Box 14.1). Remember the aim of creating any teaching materials is to help make the learning more effective and efficient.

Box 14.1 **CREATE guidelines**

C – convenience
R – relevance
E – evidence-based
A – actively involving the learner
T – technology
E – evaluating the educational impact

C is for convenience

Teaching materials must be easily accessible for the learner (Figure 14.1), particularly with the shift towards more independent learning. For convenience, learning materials need to be student centred, enabling learners to direct themselves through the material without the need for a tutor. In addition, the workplace is increasingly being used as a learning environment; so doctors need to be able to access resources in a timely manner to enhance safe practice. Convenience also applies to the teacher creating the materials, and teachers need to be wary of being too ambitious in terms of what they can produce.

To be accessible,

- materials need to be easy to read
  - ensure plenty of white space;
  - do not overload slides/web pages with too much text;
  - keep style of material uniform so that focus is on content.
- materials need to be understandable
  - think of level of learner;
  - be aware of learners' needs.
- amount of material presented need to be learner sensitive.

R is for relevance

Learners need to understand the relevance of the teaching they are receiving both for their immediate learning needs and in relation

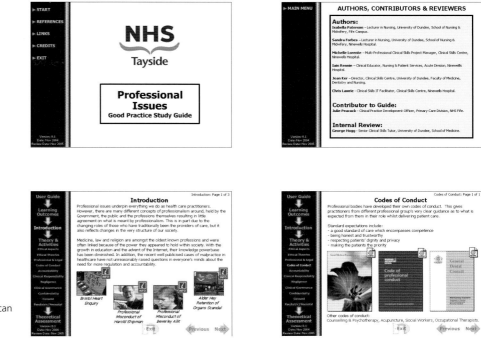

Figure 14.1 Convenience: use of e-learning can facilitate learning through flexible access via the web.

to their curricular programme. Links to other learning events can be made explicitly in the materials.

Learning materials for adult learners must cater for different learning needs and styles. Creating learning materials to meet a range of learner needs in different health care professions is challenging. This can perhaps be addressed by providing access to core material with optional content that is profession specific.

Since many students are visual learners, providing colour pictures with relevant content will be more effective.

Combining different teaching materials can also provide added relevance for the learner. For example, linking a simulated scenario about a patient with chest pain to an e-learning resource about the pathophysiology of ischaemic heart disease reinforces the link between theory and practice.

E is for evidence base

Health-care practice is constantly changing and this presents a challenge to ensure that teaching materials are up to date, especially when they relate to changes in medical practice. The Cochrane database provides systematic reviews and Pubmed can identify the latest published research in a clinical area.

In addition, there are well-recognised evidence-based guidelines which can be accessed:

SIGN guidelines – www.sign.ac.uk
NICE guidelines – www.nice.org.uk

The advent of revalidation will require all medical practitioners to provide evidence of their continuing professional development. In the case of medical teachers, tutors and facilitators this will also necessitate the need to provide up to date evidence not only of the content of their session but also of the structure of their teaching materials.

Medical education is increasingly developing an evidence base in relation to teaching materials and resources as demonstrated below by a selection of the Best Evidence-Based Medical Education (BEME) reviews (www.bemecollaboration.org).

BEME reviews include the following:

- BEME Guide No 4 – features and uses of high-fidelity medical simulations that lead to effective learning: a BEME systematic review
- BEME Guide No 6 – how can experience in clinical and community settings contribute to early medical education? A BEME systematic review
- BEME Guide No 8 – a systematic review of faculty development initiatives designed to improve teaching effectiveness in medical education
- BEME Guide No 9 – a best evidence systematic review on inter-professional education
- BEME Guide No 10 – a systematic review of the literature on the effectiveness of self-assessment in clinical education

A is for actively involving the learner

Actively involving the learner through the effective use of teaching materials will enhance deep rather than superficial learning (see Box 14.2). This can be achieved at the start of a session by:

- thinking of single questions to pose to learners;
- linking examples to learner's previous experience.

For example, when creating teaching materials such as an interactive reflective log diary in an outpatient clinic, the use of structured questions in relation to the consultation will actively engage the learner rather than just observing the consultation. This reflective

LIBRARY
EDUCATION CENTRE
PRINCESS ROYAL HOSPITAL

Box 14.2 Gagne's Nine Events of Instruction as applied to the creation of teaching materials

1. Gain attention
2. Inform the learner of the outcomes
3. Stimulate recall of previous relevant learning
4. Present the new learning
5. Provide learning guidance
6. Elicit performance (make learning materials interactive)
7. Provide feedback to ensure standards
8. Assess
9. Enhance retention and transfer

Data from: Gagne RM, Briggs LJ, Wager WF. *Principles of Instructional Design.* Wadsworth, 1985.

---

log may be kept electronically using a hand-held computer and can form the trigger material for a further teaching session at the end of the clinic.

In addition, handouts of a PowerPoint presentation following a lecture can have some self-assessment questions, which in turn can become teaching materials for a follow-up session. This iterative use of teaching materials helps to integrate learning and facilitates the transformation of learning from the classroom to the workplace. Simulation exercises as a teaching resource have been shown to be an effective tool for shortening training times in the development of technical skills (Kneebone *et al.* 2003).

T is for technology

Technology is being used increasingly by students and teachers at all levels of medical education for communication and to provide learning materials for both the informal and formal curriculum. Wikis, blogs and discussion boards provide different mediums for sharing learning and exploring understanding in an interactive dynamic way without the constraints of the classroom. Technological improvements now mean that the constraints of slow downloading and difficult access are being resolved.

When you think of technology you must think of the following:

- What added value will technology bring to achieving the learning outcomes?
- What ongoing support maintenance will the materials require?
- Will the technology require specialist hardware capacity?

There is increasing evidence that technology can enhance teaching and learning as it can facilitate active engagement in the process. Many medical schools and higher education institutes now use VLEs to deliver distance learning (Cook 2002).

Examples of available technology are as follows:

1. Second life (www.secondlife.com)
   This provides the opportunity for teachers to create a virtual workplace environment and explore consequences of actions with students without impacting on patient care. Teachers and students can create teaching materials in partnership.
2. Simulators
   Simulators are useful resources in creating realistic, safe learning environments.

3. Concept map tools
   A number of software tools are available for creating concept or mind maps. Two well known ones are Inspiration (www.inspiration.com) and CMap (http://cmap.ihmc.us).

'Reviews of E learning' provides helpful summaries of publications on research in e-learning (www.elearning-reviews.org/).

E is for educational impact

The educational impact of teaching materials enables teachers to set explicit standards in relation to both quality and content of the teaching materials. There are national quality standards for the development of online materials, and university quality assurance processes create a framework for reviewing teaching standards, including the use of teaching materials.

Kirkpatrick (1994) identified four levels of evaluating educational interventions which range from satisfaction, to learning, to behaviour change, to improved patient outcomes.

When creating new teaching materials, it is essential to obtain feedback on their usefulness and effectiveness in relationship to learning. There are different approaches to receiving feedback on teaching materials or resources. For example, feedback on clinical skills can be from patients, from the simulator and through a debriefing process from both the learner and the teacher. For other materials, focus groups involving the learners or a short questionnaire will suffice.

Using CREATE to getting started

Why are teaching materials needed?

The CREATE principles that apply here are:

- relevance
- actively involving the learner
- educational impact.

In getting started, the purpose of creating teaching materials can be addressed through three questions which relate to three CREATE guiding principles.

1. Who are the learners?
   ○ Undergraduates/junior or senior postgraduates/CPD participants
2. What are the learning outcomes related to?
   ○ knowledge skills or attitudes
   ○ health or disease process
   ○ long-term conditions
   ○ rare emergency scenarios
3. Where will the teaching materials be used?
   ○ lecture/small group/clinical setting

What are the different mediums that can be used to create teaching materials?

The CREATE principles that apply here are:

- convenience
- technology.

Many mediums can be used to create teaching materials. For example, study guides are aids to support student learning in either paper or electronic form and can assist in management of student e-learning, provide a directed focus for student activities or provide information on specific topic areas.

The following lists identify different mediums that can best be used in different teaching contexts using two CREATE guiding principles.

For lectures

- Interactive whiteboard
- Paper handouts
- PowerPoint
- Interactive PowerPoint
- Simulation role play
- Web-based activity
- Video clips

For small-group sessions

- Paper scenarios as triggers
- U-tube or other online sites as a source of film triggers for identified learning outcomes
- Anonymised patient data

For clinical settings

- Simulation exercises
  - part task trainers
  - simulated patients
  - virtual reality
  - mid-fidelity and high-fidelity simulators
- Ward or theatre settings
  - patient stories
  - critical incidents
- Community setting
  - video consultation and debrief
  - checklists

For self-directed learning

- Podcast
- Web resources
- Online resource pack on VLE
- Second life or online simulation exercise

Who should create teaching resources?

The CREATE principles that apply here are:

- evidence base
- actively involving the learner
- educational impact.

All medical teachers have both evidence-based clinical expertise and experience of teaching in the workplace. It is important to recognise the level of educational expertise required to produce evidence-based effective materials. Both educational and technological expertise may be required to develop quality teaching materials. For example, when developing an e-portfolio medical, educational and IT expertise is likely to be required. Learners can also be a useful resource in preparing teaching materials not only

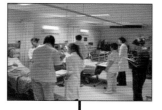 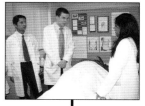

Ward simulation exercise
One of the challenges in creating resources for bedside teaching is linking the opportunistic learning from patients with the systematic and structured curriculum An e-learning package which links clinical problems with basic sciences may be useful preparation for a simulated ward exercise

Small group peer learning
It may be appropriate to have a standard paper study guide to ensure all students cover the same learning outcomes.

Figure 14.2 Technology: can be used to enhance and reinforce learning in different contexts.

for themselves but also for future groups. In addition, educational networks can provide a framework for access and development of effective resources.

What influences the creation of effective learning materials?

The two CREATE principles that apply here are:

- evidence base
- technology.

The creation of effective teaching materials is dependent on a number of factors.

1 The teacher
The time required to develop quality materials should not be underestimated. Some teachers such as skills facilitators may have time built into their job plan to develop quality evidence-based teaching materials, while others such as peer tutors or service clinicians may have to create teaching materials within their limited teaching sessions. Be realistic about the time you have available.
2 The content of the teaching materials
Some content areas lend themselves to the use of technology (Figure 14.2); for example, animation of the cardiac cycle.
3 Where the teaching is taking place

Helpful Hints

See Table 14.1.

A final thought

A systematic review of the impact of printed materials in 2005 (Freemantle *et al.*) suggested that there was little impact of printed materials on clinical practice and that more influence comes from

Table 14.1 Common pitfalls when developing effective teaching materials.

Common pitfalls
Seeing the resource as an end point, not as a means to facilitate learning
Using high-tech gizmos which can mask a positive learning experience
Not verifying that e-learning resources conform to standards
Not checking transferability of Internet resources to a learning event
Using too many attention-raising features with technology
Using humour inappropriately
Being unaware of cultural influences on learning
Overwhelming learners with numerous learning outcomes
Over highlighting learning points
Using pictures which are ambiguous in terms of meaning
Using different, distracting formatting styles
Using dense text

opinion leaders and educational visits to the workplace. This is an overt challenge to all of us to ensure teaching materials are well created for an appropriate purpose and context.

Further reading

Gagne RM. *The Conditions of Learning*. 4th ed. New York: Holt Rinehart and Winston, 1985.

Laidlaw JM, Harden RM. What is … … a study guide? *Medical Teacher* 1990; 12:7–12.

References

Cook J. The role of the virtual learning environments in UK medical education LTSN. *Bioscience Bulletin* 2002; 5 http://bio.ltsn.ac.uk.

Freemantle N, Harvey EL, Wolf F, Grimshaw JM, Grilli R, Bero LA. Printed educational materials: effects on professional practice and health care outcomes. *The Cochrane database of systematic reviews*. The Cochrane library, The Cochrane Collaboration. 2005;3

Kirkpatrick DL. *Evaluating Training Programmes: The Four Levels*. San Francisco, CA: Berrett–Koehler Publishers, 1994.

Kneebone RL, Nestel D, Moorthy K, Taylor P, Bann S, Munz Y, Darzi A. Learning the skills of flexible sigmoidoscopy – the wider perspective. *Medical Education* 2003;37(suppl 1):50–80.

CHAPTER 15

Learning and Teaching Professionalism

Sylvia R. Cruess and Richard L. Cruess

McGill University, Montreal, Quebec, Canada

OVERVIEW

- Professionalism should be taught explicitly throughout the medical curriculum
- The two major components of teaching professionalism are
  - explicit teaching of the cognitive base
  - stage-appropriate opportunities for experiential learning and reflection throughout the curriculum
- The professionalism of both students and faculty must be evaluated
- Faculty development in the teaching and modelling of professionalism is essential to ensure adequate implementation of a programme

Introduction

This chapter will emphasise the importance of (i) being explicit about the teaching of professionalism, (ii) defining the content of professionalism courses, (iii) designing appropriate assessment strategies and (iv) agreeing on the principles which underpin the design and implementation of professionalism programmes. The design of a professionalism programme does not differ from designing a programme in any other aspect of medicine. The principles of instructional design apply just as they do to the rest of the medical curriculum. As always, the essential steps are to establish the goals and objectives of the programme, develop the content, choose the methods which will best encourage learning and assess what has been learnt. Assessment is not only about measuring student achievement; it is also about evaluating whether the goals and objectives of the programme have been achieved.

Why must physicians learn professionalism?

The formal teaching of professionalism in medicine has a relatively short history and only recently has become a requirement. In earlier times, the practice, organisation and funding of health care was

ABC of Learning and Teaching in Medicine, 2nd edition.
Edited by Peter Cantillon and Diana Wood. © 2010 Blackwell Publishing Ltd.

much simpler and less threatening to professional values. As a result, it was possible for the attitudes and behaviours expected of the ideal physician to be passed from generation to generation by respected role models. While the role modelling associated with the classical approach to professional apprenticeship remains an extremely powerful tool, it alone is no longer sufficient. The threats to professionalism are sufficiently great that it must be taught explicitly at all levels.

What must be learnt

Determining the cognitive base (core knowledge of the nature of contemporary professionalism, its history and evolution, and the reasons for its existence in society) is often so difficult that many programmes neglect to take this essential first step. In the absence of a stated cognitive base, including a definition, the concept of professionalism remains indistinct for students, the reasons for the presence of professional obligations not fully understood and the relationship between teaching and assessment is not logical. It follows, therefore, that the initial challenge in developing a professionalism programme is to agree upon a definition consistent with the literature on professionalism so that faculty and students share the same understanding and use the same vocabulary.

The literature is replete with definitions, most of which are quite similar. Box 15.1 contains a definition that was developed specifically for use in teaching. Its disadvantage is its length, but its strength is that it is inclusive and can serve as the basis for discussion of the issues surrounding professionalism.

An agreed definition provides the basis for an outline of the characteristics of a professional. Physicians in their day to day practice function simultaneously as both healers and professionals, and most definitions include both roles. For teaching purposes, it is helpful to separate them. This step can be justified, because the two roles have different histories and have evolved independently, although in parallel. All societies have required healers who minister to the sick. The traditions of the healer in the Western world are derived from Hellenic Greece with the Hippocratic and Aesculapian traditions. Curing arrived relatively late with the advent of scientific medicine. While the word profession is ancient, the modern professions whose origins are in the guilds and universities of medieval Europe and England arose in the middle of the nineteenth century

Box 15.1 **A definition of profession for medical educators**

Profession – An occupation whose core element is work, based upon the mastery of a complex body of knowledge and skills. It is a vocation in which knowledge of some department of science or learning, or the practice of an art founded upon it, is used in the service of others. Its members are governed by codes of ethics and profess a commitment to competence, integrity and morality, altruism and the promotion of the public good within their domain. These commitments form the basis of a social contract between a profession and society, which in return grants the profession a monopoly over the use of its knowledge base, the right to considerable autonomy in practice and to an important role in regulation. Professions and their members are accountable to those being served, to society and to the profession.

when licensing laws granted a monopoly over practice to the medical profession. Each role has its traditional duties and obligations, many of which overlap.

Figure 15.1 includes a list (derived from the literature) of the characteristics of the physician, including those of the healer, of the professional and those shared by both. These attributes form the basis of societal expectations of physicians, and hence should serve as the core of teaching about the nature of professionalism. Students, faculty and practising physicians must understand these attributes and demonstrate them in their daily lives. It must be stressed that what both patients and society require are the services of the healer. Professionalism is used as the means of organising these services. Society grants professionals autonomy in practice, an important role in regulation, privileged status and financial rewards on the understanding that the profession will assure the competence of its members, be altruistic, demonstrate morality and

integrity in their day to day lives and address issues of concern to society. This is the essence of medicine's social contract from which is derived medicine's obligations to society. If individual physicians or the profession fail to meet society's legitimate expectations, the social contract will be altered, with a consequent change in medicine's professional status. Presenting professionalism in this context to students at all levels provides a coherent base for medicine's professional obligations, along with cogent reasons for meeting them.

A few attributes require emphasis. Clinical competence is the essential foundation of being a health professional, but caring and compassion, openness, respect for the patient's dignity and autonomy and that elusive term 'presence' (accompanying the patient throughout the course of their illness) are essential to fulfilling the healer role. Patients must be able to trust their physicians and to believe that they will be altruistic, placing the patient's needs above their own. Physicians must retain sufficient autonomy so that they and their patients together can make evidence-based decisions about treatment without external interference. Finally, the physician's role in the regulatory process must be taught and learnt. No matter who is responsible for quality control and discipline, the setting and maintenance of standards for education, training and practice will remain an essential function of the profession. Students must learn this at an early stage of their education and understand the consequences if the profession fails to meet this obligation.

How should it be taught?

Professionalism's cognitive base should be introduced formally early in the curriculum and should appear with increasing levels of complexity on a regular basis throughout undergraduate and postgraduate education. It is not sufficient to give one or two lectures and assume that the issue has been addressed. It must be taught and learnt explicitly so that it is understood by all. The cognitive base is much more than knowledge about professionalism. It also should include the value system of medicine which must be internalised by all physicians during the long process of socialisation which transforms members of the lay public into true professionals. Explicit measures must be taken to ensure that this internalisation takes place.

The cognitive base of professionalism should be taught throughout the continuum of medical education (Box 15.2).

Learning the cognitive base can be facilitated through lectures (to provide frameworks, definitions and stimulate curiosity), small groups (to explore personal interpretations and biases), problem-based learning or collaborative learning formats using case studies as the stimulus. Every physician must understand the nature of professionalism, its role in sustaining medicine's relationship to society, the obligations necessary to maintain this relationship and the consequences of failing to meet these obligations.

However, focusing on the cognitive base alone is not sufficient. Since professional identity arises 'from a long term combination of experience and reflection on experience' (Hilton and Slotnick 2005), the learner must be provided with stage-appropriate opportunities to experience the challenges and dilemmas faced by practising physicians and to reflect upon these events in the context

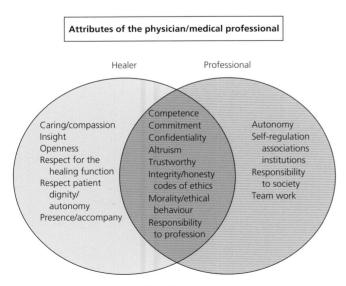

Attributes of the physician/medical professional

Healer   Professional

Caring/compassion
Insight
Openness
Respect for the
  healing function
Respect patient
  dignity/
  autonomy
Presence/accompany

Competence
Commitment
Confidentiality
Altruism
Trustworthy
Integrity/honesty
  codes of ethics
Morality/ethical
  behaviour
Responsibility
  to profession

Autonomy
Self-regulation
  associations
  institutions
Responsibility
  to society
Team work

Figure 15.1 The attributes traditionally associated with the healer are shown in the left hand circle and those with the professional on the right. As can be seen, there are attributes unique to each role. Those shared by both are found in the large area of overlap of the circles. This list of attributes is drawn from the literature on healing and professionalism.

LIBRARY
EDUCATION CENTRE
PRINCESS ROYAL HOSPITAL

Box 15.2 **Methods of teaching professionalism**

The cognitive base	Experiential learning and reflection
Lectures	Real-life clinical experience
Small-group instruction	Simulated clinical experience
Inclusion in cases for problem-based learning	Clinical vignettes
	from general experience
Review of the literature on professionalism	from the learner's experience
	Video clips
	Narratives
	personal
	literature or films
	Role play
	Other

All must be accompanied by time for reflection in a safe environment

---

of being a professional (Box 15.2). A conscious effort must be made to ensure that all learners have an opportunity to experience real or simulated situations in which they must evaluate their own professional values and act upon them. Real-life clinical situations are obviously the most powerful, but not all students can be exposed to all aspects of professionalism in this way. Small-group discussions involving case vignettes, video clips, narratives, role-plays or other educational methods should be structured so that the many sides of professionalism are experienced (Boxes 15.3 and 15.4). Learners must then be encouraged to reflect often upon these experiences in a safe environment so that the process of reflection becomes habitual. Role models have an extremely important part to play in this process. The role models must understand professionalism and its attributes and be able to stimulate reflection on the pertinent aspects of professionalism being modelled. They have the ability to consciously model exemplary professional behaviour. Unfortunately, professional role models can also display unprofessional behaviour, a leading cause of the well-documented cynicism which can develop in some students. A key question for anyone planning a professionalism programme is what to do about managing the exposure of medical students to negative role models.

Assessing professionalism

Box 15.5 outlines the most common methods used to assess professionalism. Four points require emphasis. In the first place, the definition chosen, along with the attributes of the professional, should dictate what is being assessed. Second, the learner's knowledge of the nature of contemporary professionalism should be evaluated using robust methods including written examinations, MCQ's and so on. Third, the performance of the learners, including observed professional or unprofessional behaviour, should be evaluated using multiple evaluators and multiple techniques to ensure greater reliability. Finally, the professionalism of faculty members must also be evaluated in order to ensure that the learning environment supports rather than subverts the teaching of professionalism.

Box 15.3 **Example of the use of a vignette to promote reflection**

The objective: To promote discussion on the role of the physician in regulation.
One solution: In small groups discuss the following vignette:
You are a final year medical student working in a medical outpatient clinic in a teaching hospital. The clinician responsible for the clinic has slurred speech and smells of alcohol.
Issues to discuss: caring and compassion, morality and ethical behaviour, self-regulation, responsibility to society, responsibility to the profession.

Box 15.4 **Example of the use of a video clip to promote reflection**

The objective: To promote discussion on altruism.
One solution: In small groups discuss a video showing the following:
A cardiologist is about to leave the hospital early to watch his daughter perform in the finals of a gymnastic competition. He is informed that a patient whom he has treated previously for a myocardial infarction is in the emergency room with chest pain and has requested that he treat him.
Issues to discuss: altruism, lifestyle, caring and compassion, commitment, teamwork.

Box 15.5 **Methods for evaluating professionalism**

Evaluating knowledge of the cognitive base

Multiple-choice questions
Short answer questions
Essays
Independent research projects
Portfolios

Evaluating professional performance

Multiple observations by multiple observers
Physician-faculty member, registrar/resident
Other health professional
Patient
Peers
OSCE
Critical incident reports
Professionalism Mini-Evaluation Exercise (P-MEX)
Portfolios
Other

Implementing a programme

The teaching of professionalism should permeate all aspects of the education of the physician of the future. Implementing such a programme crosses departmental lines, is necessary at the undergraduate and postgraduate levels and will certainly be a requirement of the continuing professional development of the future. Successful programmes share several characteristics. Strong and visible institutional leadership is essential and is usually expressed by the allocation of both curricular time and resources to the programme. Responsibility for a professionalism programme is usually given to a broad-based committee chaired by a knowledgeable individual who serves as the programme's champion. Attention needs to be given to the teaching environment that should support and reward professional behaviour and not tolerate unprofessional activities. Role models, who can have such a positive or negative impact on learners, must be recognised and rewarded when appropriate. If their performance is unsatisfactory, they must be offered remediation or removed from contact with students. Virtually all successful professionalism programmes have established faculty development programmes on teaching and assessing professionalism and on role modelling.

Professionalism should be taught throughout the continuum of medical education. While the depth of knowledge about professionalism will vary depending upon the level of the learner, the essentials of professionalism will not change. There should, therefore, be continuity between undergraduate and postgraduate professionalism programmes. Finally, it is not necessary to institute a complete programme at one time. Once an overall design has been agreed upon, it can be implemented incrementally as each unit is developed.

As has been stated by the Royal College of Physicians of London (2005), 'medical professionalism lies at the heart of being a good doctor'. For this reason, the successful design and implementation of programmes to teach and evaluate professionalism are essential if teaching establishments in medicine are to meet their professional obligations to society.

Further reading

ABIM (American Board of Internal Medicine) Foundation. ACP (American College of Physicians) Foundation. European Federation of Internal Medicine. Medical professionalism in the new millennium: a physician charter. *Annals of Internal Medicine* 2002;136:243–246; *Lancet* 359:520–523.

Cruess RL, Cruess SR, Steinert Y. (Eds). *Teaching Medical Professionalism*. New York: Cambridge University Press, 2009.

Steinert Y, Cruess RL, Cruess SR, Boudreau JD, Fuks A. Faculty development as an instrument of change: a case study on teaching professionalism. *Academic Medicine* 2007;82:1057–1010.

References

Hilton SR, Slotnick HB. Proto-professionalism: how professionalization occurs across the continuum of medical education. *Medical Education* 2005; 39:58–65.

Royal College of Physicians of London. *Doctors in Society: Medical Professionalism in a Changing World*. London, UK: Royal College of Physicians of London, 2005.

CHAPTER 16

Making It All Happen: Faculty Development for Busy Teachers

Yvonne Steinert

McGill University, Montreal, Quebec, Canada

OVERVIEW

- Faculty development, or staff development as it is often called, aims to help teachers develop the skills relevant to their institutional and faculty position

- Faculty development programmes and activities can transmit new knowledge and skills, reinforce or alter beliefs about teaching, provide a conceptual framework for what is often performed on an intuitive basis and introduce clinicians to a community of teachers

- Faculty development includes *all* activities that teachers pursue to improve their teaching skills in both *individual* and *group* settings

- *Individual approaches* to faculty development include learning on-the-job, observing role models in action and reflecting on teaching and learning. *Group approaches* include structured faculty development activities such as workshops or longitudinal programmes, work-based learning and belonging to a community of teachers

- To make faculty development work for you, it is important to identify your needs, determine your preferred method(s) of learning and choose a programme (or activity) that works for you. Finding a mentor and a community of teachers that support your vision and your goals can also be extremely beneficial

---

What is faculty development?

Faculty development, or staff development as it is often called, refers to that broad range of activities institutions use to *renew* or *assist* teachers in their multiple roles (Centra 1978). That is, the goal of faculty development is to help faculty members acquire the skills relevant to their institutional and faculty position, and to sustain their vitality, both now and in the future. Although faculty development often refers to a planned programme designed to prepare teachers for their multiple roles, clinicians often engage in both formal and informal 'faculty development' to enhance their

knowledge and skills. For the purpose of this discussion, faculty development will refer to all activities teachers pursue to improve their teaching skills in both *individual* and *group* settings.

Why is faculty development important?

Faculty development designed to improve teaching effectiveness can provide clinicians with new knowledge and skills about teaching and learning. It can also reinforce or alter attitudes or beliefs about teaching, provide a conceptual framework for what is often performed intuitively and introduce clinicians to a community of teachers (Steinert 2010a). As the expectations of teachers and demands for accountability in higher education increase, the need for professional development will proliferate. It is ironic that most physicians, while experts in their field, have had little or no training in how to teach.

Common faculty development goals and content areas

Comprehensive faculty development includes both individual and organisational development. At the *individual* level, faculty development can address *attitudes and beliefs* about teaching and learning; transmit *knowledge* about educational principles and instructional design; and develop *skills* in teaching, curriculum design and educational leadership. At the *organisational* level, it can help to create opportunities for learning; recognise and reward excellence in teaching and learning; and address systems issues that impede effective educational practices (Steinert 2010b).

To date, the majority of faculty development programmes have focused on teaching improvement, with a particular emphasis on clinical teaching, small-group facilitation, feedback and evaluation. A number of activities also target specific core competencies (e.g. the teaching and evaluation of communication skills) and the use of technology in teaching and learning; however, less attention has been paid to personal development, educational leadership and scholarship and organisational development and change. Yet without organisational change, new knowledge and skills may be difficult to implement. Clinical teachers should choose their faculty development activities wisely so that their perceived needs and goals can be met.

ABC of Learning and Teaching in Medicine, 2nd edition.
Edited by Peter Cantillon and Diana Wood. © 2010 Blackwell Publishing Ltd.

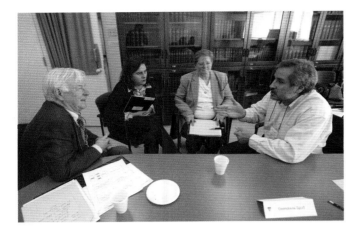

Individual approaches to faculty development

You become adept at what you do by the nature of your responsibilities and by learning on the spot . . .

Learning from experience

Prior to engaging in organised faculty development programmes, teachers often learn through 'on-the-job training', by the nature of their responsibilities, observing their colleagues in action or reflecting on their experiences. Some have said that educational leadership roles in medical education offer 'laboratories' in which to experiment with new methods and ideas; others have noted that they learn through role modelling or critically thinking about what they are doing. The role of reflection in clinical medicine, and the notion of *reflection in action* and *reflection on action*, has received increasing attention in recent years. This process of self-assessment and critical analysis is equally important in faculty development, as reflection on teaching allows for the integration of theoretical concepts into practice, greater learning through experience and enhanced critical thinking and judgement (Box 16.1).

Box 16.1 **Reflection on teaching and learning**

You need to do more than simply teach . . . You need to reflect on your teaching, discuss your teaching with other educators, and try to analyze and improve what you are doing.

- Reflection *in* action – while performing an act/role, analysing what is being done
- Reflection *on* action – after performing the act/role, reflecting on the impact of the action on the student and yourself
- Reflection *for* action – reflecting on what has been learnt for the future

Adapted from: Schön (1983) and Lachman and Pawlina (2006)

Learning from peers and students

Learning from experience can be heightened by peer and student feedback. Although teachers are often reluctant to solicit the views of others, it can be extremely helpful to ask a colleague to observe you and provide feedback after a specific teaching encounter; it can be equally beneficial to discuss a recent challenge or critical incident. Peer coaching, as this activity is sometimes called, has particular appeal for clinicians because it occurs in the practice setting, enables individualised learning and fosters collaboration (Orlander *et al.* 2000).

Soliciting student feedback can be equally beneficial, and in fact, a few concise questions can trigger useful discussions (Box 16.2). Moreover, an appreciative review of student evaluations can provide useful information, especially if teachers view these observations and comments as opportunities for learning. In multiple ways, engaging in dialogue with students and peers can help clinical teachers to break down complex teaching activities into understandable components, link intent, behaviour and educational outcomes, facilitate the examination of personal assumptions and examine the effectiveness of specific teaching practices (Steinert 2010b).

Box 16.2 **Soliciting feedback from students and peers**

Questions to solicit feedback from students and peers

- What did you learn in this teaching encounter?
- What about this encounter was helpful to you? What was not?
- What could I have done differently to make it more useful?

Questions to consider when reviewing student evaluations

- Is there a pattern that runs across diverse evaluations?
- What am I doing well? What might I do differently?
- How can I use this as an opportunity for learning about myself?

Learning from experience as well as peers and students can be further augmented by independent study, online learning and guided reading. In fact, numerous print and web-based resources (Box 16.3) are available to inform and support clinical teachers.

Box 16.3 **A sample of medical education journals (Steinert 2005)**

Academic Medicine	www.academicmedicine.org
Advances in Health Sciences Education	www.springer.com/
Journal for Continuing Education in the Health Professions	www.jcehp.com
Medical Education	www.blackwell-science.com
Medical Teacher	www.medicalteacher.org
Pédagogie Médicale	www.pedagogie-medicale.org
Teaching & Learning in Medicine	www.siumed.edu/tlm

Finding a mentor can also help to enhance independent learning, as mentors can provide direction or support, help to understand the organisational culture and introduce teachers to invaluable professional networks.

Group approaches to faculty development

Participating in a faculty development workshop gives me a sense of community, self-awareness, motivation and validation of current practices and beliefs.

Structured faculty development activities

Common faculty development formats include workshops and seminars, short courses, fellowships, advanced degrees and longitudinal programmes.

Workshop, seminars and short courses

Workshops are popular because of their inherent flexibility and promotion of active learning. Of varying duration, they are commonly used to promote skill acquisition or help teachers to prepare for curricular change. Although transfer to the workplace is sometimes challenging, they can also help to develop expertise in curricular design and innovation (Box 16.4).

Box 16.4 **A selection of common faculty development topics (Steinert 2005)**

- Teaching when there is no time to teach
- Actions speak louder than words: promoting interaction in teaching
- Learning is not a spectator sport: effective small-group teaching
- Advanced clinical teaching skills
- Teaching in the ambulatory setting
- Teaching technical and procedural skills
- Giving feedback: tell it like it is?
- Evaluating residents: truth or consequences?
- The 'problem' student: whose problem is it?
- Teaching and evaluating professionalism

Fellowships and degree programmes

Fellowships and degree programmes are becoming increasingly popular in many settings. Most universities in the United Kingdom now require faculty members to undertake a certificate in teaching and learning and many medical schools provide fellowship opportunities for advanced training. These programmes can be particularly useful to individuals interested in educational leadership and scholarship.

Longitudinal programmes

Integrated longitudinal programmes, such as a *Teaching Scholars Programme*, have been developed as an alternative to fellowship or degree programmes. These programmes, which allow teachers to

continue to practice and teach while improving their educational knowledge and skills, can also encourage the development of leadership and scholarly activity in medical education.

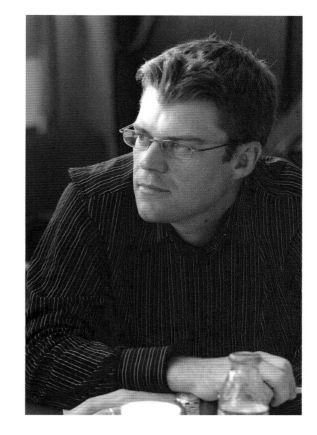

Work-based learning

Work-based learning has been defined as learning *for* work, learning *at* work and learning *from* work (Swanwick 2008). This concept, which is closely tied to the notion of community, is fundamental to the development of clinical teachers for whom 'learning on-the-job' is often the first entry into teaching. Moreover, as learning usually takes place in the workplace, where teachers conduct their clinical, research and teaching activities, it is important to view these everyday experiences as 'learning experiences'.

Becoming a member of a teaching community

Clinical teachers often note the benefits of working together with a network of committed colleagues. As a junior colleague observed, 'If you are able to immerse yourself in a group, it gives you so much. If you start with some experience, and you mix yourself into a group with like interests, you get much more out of it . . . especially as you begin to look at things critically with education glasses on' (Steinert 2010b). This quote underscores the benefit of *valuing* and *finding* community, as in many ways, sharing a common vision and language – and becoming a member of a community of teachers – can be a critical step in faculty development.

LIBRARY
EDUCATION CENTRE
PRINCESS ROYAL HOSPITAL

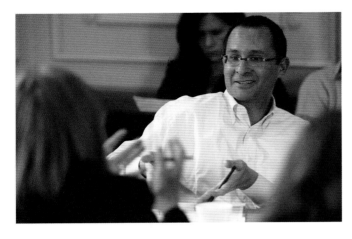

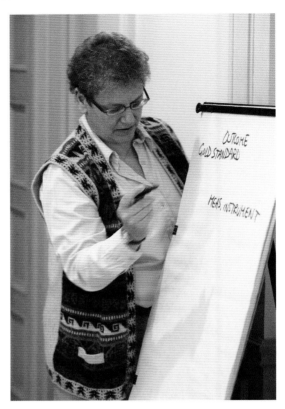

Does faculty development make a difference?

In 2006, as part of the BEME (Best Evidence in Medical Education) collaboration, an international group of medical educators systematically reviewed the faculty development literature to ascertain the impact of formal initiatives on teaching improvement. The results of this review indicated overall satisfaction with faculty development programmes. Moreover, participants found programmes to be useful, acceptable and relevant to their objectives and they valued the methods used. Teachers also reported positive changes in attitudes toward faculty development *and* teaching as a result of their involvement in these activities and cited a greater awareness of personal strengths and limitations, increased motivation and enthusiasm for teaching and learning, and a notable appreciation of the benefits of professional development. In addition, they reported increased knowledge of educational principles and strategies and gains in teaching skills.

The BEME review also highlighted specific features that contribute to the effectiveness of formal faculty development activities. These 'key features' incorporated the role of experiential learning and the importance of applying what had been learnt; the provision of feedback; effective peer relationships, which included the value of role modelling, exchange of information and collegial support; well-designed interventions that followed principles of teaching and learning; and the use of multiple instructional methods to achieve intended objectives. Awareness of these components can help teachers to choose effective programmes.

Making faculty development work for you

Both formal and informal approaches, in individual and group settings, can facilitate personal and professional development as a teacher. Irrespective of which approach works for you, it is important to identify your needs, determine your preferred method(s) of learning and choose a programme (or activity) that works for you. Finding a mentor and a community of teachers that support your vision and your goals can also be extremely helpful.

Identify your needs

The following attributes and behaviours of effective clinical teachers have been identified in the literature: enthusiasm, a positive attitude towards teaching, rapport with students and patients, availability and accessibility, clinical competence and subject matter expertise. Core teaching skills have also been identified: the establishment of a positive learning environment; the setting of clear objectives and expectations; the provision of timely and relevant information; the effective use of questioning and other instructional methods; appropriate role modelling; and the provision of constructive feedback and objective-based evaluations. Take time to assess your strengths and areas for improvement and consider how you might improve your teaching abilities.

Determine your preferred method(s) of learning

As adults, we all have preferred methods of learning. Some of us prefer to learn on our own and others prefer to learn with colleagues, in a formal or informal setting. Think about your preferred method(s) and build this into your faculty development plan.

Choose a programme that works for you

As previously described, numerous activities can facilitate teaching improvement. Choose an activity that is pertinent to your needs and preferred method of learning and that will help you to achieve your teaching and learning goals. At times, independent learning in an informal setting will be most appropriate for you. At other times, a structured activity (such as a workshop or short course) will be most pertinent.

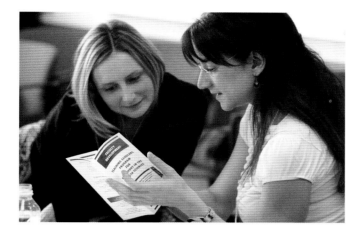

Identify a mentor or guide

Clinical teachers frequently comment on the role of mentors in their personal development, as they value their support, their ability to challenge personal assumptions and their assistance in framing a vision for the future. Whenever possible, find someone who can help to fulfil this role and provide guidance as you try to improve as a teacher and identify a faculty development approach that will work for you.

Find a community of teachers

As stated earlier, a community of teachers can help you to refine your vision, develop your skills and find ways to improve as a teacher. It has often been said that teaching is a 'team sport'. We must remember that achieving educational excellence cannot be accomplished independently and we must try to find – and value – a community of like-minded individuals.

Conclusion

The Dutch term for faculty development, *Docentprofessionalisering*, loosely translates as the 'professionalisation of teaching'. In many ways, engaging in faculty development, either individually or as part of a group, is the first step to the professionalisation of teaching in medical education.

Further reading

Hesketh E, Bagnall G, Buckley E, Friedman M, Goodall E, Harden R, Laidlaw J, Leighton-Beck L, McKinlay P, Newton R, Oughton R. A framework for developing excellence as a clinical educator. *Medical Education* 2001;35(6):555–564.

Irby D. What clinical teachers in medicine need to know. *Academic Medicine* 1994;69(5):333–342.

Steinert Y, Mann K, Centeno A, Dolmans D, Spencer J, Gelula M, Prideaux D. A systematic review of faculty development initiatives designed to improve teaching effectiveness in medical education: BEME Guide No. 8. *Medical Teaching* 2006;28(6):497–526.

Wenger E. *Communities of Practice: Learning, Meaning and Identity*. New York: Cambridge University Press, 1999.

Wilkerson L, Irby DM. Strategies for improving teaching practices: a comprehensive approach to faculty development. *Academic Medicine* 1998;73(4): 387–396.

References

Centra J. Types of faculty development programs. *Journal on Higher Education* 1978;49(2):151–162.

Lachman N, Pawlina W. Integrating professionalism in early medical education: the theory and application of reflective practice in the anatomy curriculum. *Clinical Anatomy* 2006;19(5):456–460.

Orlander J, Gupta M, Fincke B, Manning M, Hershman W. Co-teaching: a faculty development strategy. *Medical Education* 2000;34(4):257–65.

Schön D. *The Reflective Practitioner: How Professionals Think in Action*. New York: Basic Books, 1983.

Steinert Y. Staff development for clinical teachers. *Clinical Teaching* 2005; 2(2):104–110.

Steinert Y. Developing medical educators: A jouney, not a destination. In T. Swanwick (Ed.). *Understanding Medical Education: Evidence, Theory and Practice*. Edinburgh: Association for the Study of Medical Education, 2010 (a).

Steinert Y. Becoming a better teacher: From intuition to intent. In: J. Ende (Ed.). *Theory and Practice of Teaching Medicine*. Philadelphia: American College of Physicians, 2010 (b).

Swanwick T. See one, do one, then what? Faculty development in postgraduate medical education. *Postgraduate Medical Journal* 2008;84:339–343.

CHAPTER 17

Supporting Students in Difficulty

Dason Evans and Jo Brown

St. George's, University of London, London, UK

Our greatest glory is not in never failing, but in rising every time we fall.

– Confucius

OVERVIEW

- Supporting learners in difficulty is a fundamental professional role of a teacher
- Students struggle for a broad and complex range of reasons
- An educational assessment interview is a useful tool for identifying reasons for difficulty
- Interventions should be individualised and holistic; simple interventions can have good outcomes
- Follow-up and coordination with other providers of support is important

---

In the current educational climate, abandoning students who are struggling academically is culturally, financially and ethically unacceptable.

– Brown and Evans (2005)

Most of us will struggle or fail at something connected with learning during our working life. By overcoming these difficulties, we become better at solving future challenges and also, perhaps, develop more understanding and empathy for others. Students are no different.

Modern medicine welcomes learners from traditional and non-traditional backgrounds, graduates of other disciplines and mature learners. Students present with a variety of abilities (both intellectual and practical) and levels of maturity, differences in life experience, problem-solving and learning techniques. This diversity brings with it strengths and weaknesses in a learning context.

Supporting learners in difficulty is a fundamental professional role of a teacher. The main aim of this support is to help students develop mature, effective learning habits that will sustain them throughout their professional lives.

The job of the teacher, therefore, is to:

- recognise the presentation of a student in difficulty;
- investigate its origins thoroughly;
- come up with a diagnosis;
- facilitate strategies for overcoming problems;
- follow-up as necessary.

'During A levels I was always able to revise everything really quickly just before exams but this didn't work for me at medical school. I had to retake my second year because I failed exams on two occasions and had to learn a different way of studying for deep understanding. I think I was a late starter.' Joel – fourth year student

– taken from Evans and Brown (2009)

How do students in difficulty present?

Students who struggle present in many obvious, and sometimes less obvious, ways (Ford *et al.* 2008). Common ways are listed below.

- Failing a written or practical exam
- Poor attendance
- Issues with professionalism, for example, plagiarism, lateness, attitude and so on
- Failure to clerk and/or present patients
- Poor preparation for sessions
- Late or absent work hand in

Sometimes students can be identified by their 'separateness' from a group, or their reluctance to join in a teaching session or discussion. Students may look anxious or depressed (Box 17.1). Interestingly, other staff members will often know the student and share concerns about them.

'It used to really bother me that different consultants had different approaches to the same skill, and wanted me to do it their way. It took me ages to realise that over the years I would need to find a way that works for me.' Philip – fourth year student

– taken from Evans and Brown (2009)

ABC of Learning and Teaching in Medicine, 2nd edition.
Edited by Peter Cantillon and Diana Wood. © 2010 Blackwell Publishing Ltd.

Box 17.1 **Presentations**

Student A   Adil presented at the end of his third year, failing his written examinations but passing his OSCE with a 'B' grade. Excellent A-level results, failed one of his written exams in the second year, late with some in-course assignments

Student B   Richard was an anxious student who did quite well in written exams but was not confident in practical exams. He stayed behind after teaching to ask extra questions in order to understand everything thoroughly. He struggled to know the exact nature of each exam and did not seem to be aware of the hidden curriculum

Student C   Elizabeth, a 'grade A' student, failed her first clinical skills exam (OSCE) in the third year, passing the written exam with high marks

Student D   Tuan, an international student, was struggling with practical exams and talking to patients. His tutor was worried about his relationships with patients and by his frequent non-attendance on the wards. He was isolated from other students, lived with other international students and rarely spoke English outside of university

Student E   Louise failed the practical exam at the end of her third year. She had managed to pass her written exam. Her attendance at teaching sessions and on the wards was poor, but just about acceptable. Teachers had noticed she seemed withdrawn, but had not talked to her about this

Why do students struggle?

Students struggle for a wide and varied range of interacting reasons, with no two students presenting or reacting in the same way. Figure 17.1 represents the range of reasons identified through thematic review of the educational assessment interviews of a series of 120 students in academic difficulty, in one institution, over a 6-year-period. Each individual student commonly had issues in more than one area and the relationships between these issues were usually complex and interdependent. It follows, therefore, that it is essential to have an individualised and holistic approach to helping students in difficulty.

Perhaps counter-intuitively, many medical students with a previously good academic record seem to have difficulty with knowing how to learn effectively and efficiently. This includes students with superficial learning styles, those who have difficulty in one form or another in their study skills (including note taking, learning in the clinical environment, time management, planning learning), difficulties with planning revision, engaging with peer learning and so forth.

Mental illness, physical illness, disability and specific learning difficulties (such as dyslexia) (Box 17.2) are relatively common in the general population, and also within the medical school population (Dyrbye *et al*. 2006). These issues commonly interact with other issues (e.g. depression often linking with isolation, motivation, learning in a group).

Similarly, issues around motivation and attendance interact with many of the other issues in Figure 17.1 and cannot be accurately represented on a two-dimensional diagram.

'I really like to understand things fully. Sometimes I spend hours on one small thing, looking in the library and on the net to try and understand it completely. I ran out of time in my revision and did badly in my first year exams.' Dimitris – second year student
                                    – taken from Evans and Brown (2009)

Box 17.2 **Problem list**

Student A   Relying on an 'excellent memory', Adil had no habit of regular study but instead 'crammed' 2 weeks before the exams. The volume covered by the third year exams was just too much to cram. He was an important member of the rugby club, both on and off the field, with every evening during term time filled with social activities

Student B   Richard had a poor life–work balance and studied most evenings and all weekend. He was driven by workload and his struggle to understand everything in great depth. He was socially isolated, rarely went out for fun and never studied in a group

Student C   Having good study skills for knowledge, Elizabeth applied the same skills to learning clinical skills (focusing on book work, making notes, visualising, but not on hands-on practice or on receiving feedback). She did not have a regular habit of examining patients as she was uncomfortable with the incompetence of learning as a novice

Student D   Tuan's formal spoken English was good but he had difficulty with colloquial English and pronunciation. He had an inflexible checklist system for history taking which was robotic and impeded his ability to build relationships with patients

Student E   Louise was having difficulty concentrating, eating and sleeping and it became clear on discussion that she was clinically depressed. She was getting up at 3.00 am to do her book work in order to 'keep up'. She was miserable but had no insight into the fact that she was ill

Educational assessment interview – making an 'educational diagnosis'

It is worthwhile setting aside time to conduct a formal, focused, but friendly discussion with students to explore the possible causes of difficulty in some depth (Sayer *et al*. 2002). Sometimes this interview will be the first opportunity a student may have had to discuss learning problems.

Some useful areas to discuss:

• Presenting problem
  ○ What does the student see as the problem/s?
  ○ What do they see as the cause/s?

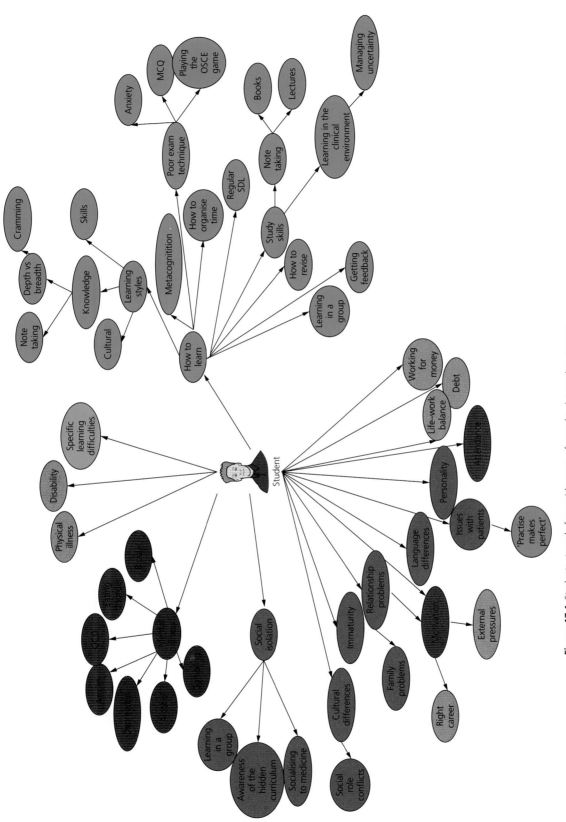

Figure 17.1 Students struggle for a wide range of complex, interacting reasons.

LIBRARY
EDUCATION CENTRE
PRINCESS ROYAL HOSPITAL

- Learning
  - How do they learn knowledge?
    - planning
    - preparation
    - revision
  - How do they learn clinical skills?
    - preparation
    - practice
    - feedback
  - How do they learn clinical communication skills?
    - preparation
    - practice
    - feedback
  - What is their study pattern?
    - Do they work regularly?
    - How many hours per week are they studying?
  - Learning with patients
    - How many patients per week are they fully clerking?
    - Are there any difficulties approaching patients?
  - How do they organise their notes/handouts/files?
  - How did they do in their written/practical exams?
- Personal situation
  - accommodation
  - relationships
  - money and so on.
- Attendance
  - What percentage would they put on their attendance?
  - What did the student attend last week?
- Motivation
  - When in their life were they most motivated to be a doctor (scale of 0–10)?
  - Where are they now on that scale (0–10)?

> 'It hit me when I had missed deadlines for 3 assignments, owed library fines of over £15.00 and couldn't face the mess in my room any more that something had to be done – something had to change. I was always trying to catch up with everyone else.' Shobna – second year student
>
> – taken from Evans and Brown (2009)

Interventions

A student-centred educational assessment interview can often act as an intervention in itself, helping the student explore the reasons for poor performance and plan how to overcome them. Interventions that are owned by the student and that target the different problem areas affecting that student seem to have most success.

Simple, targeted suggestions from tutors can often have significant effects. Such suggestions might include the following:

- Studying in the library before going home.
- Suggestions around planning regular learning, perhaps based on a simple timetable and published learning objectives.
- Practical suggestions on the importance of working with other students, and how to start a peer study group.

- Improving motivation through 'positive spirals' – for example, studying a topic which is likely to come up in clinic tomorrow (asthma management guidelines before asthma clinic) is likely to result in rewarding positive emotional response and encouragement to continue studying. Helping students realise that they can manage their own motivation in this way can be transformational.

Students may not be aware of the broad network of support available to them. Within most medical schools or their associated universities, these networks include departments providing learning support in the form of workshops, one-to-one sessions and often formal assessment by educational psychologists. Students' unions or the institution commonly provide debt and welfare advice; all medical schools will have a confidential counselling service, many with access to psychological therapies such as CBT (for depression, performance anxiety, etc.), and all students should have access to a personal tutor of one form or another.

The roles of doctor and tutor can result in conflict, and it is wise not to provide medical care for students whom you also provide academic care to. On occasion, however, it may be useful to give the student a letter for their GP if you suspect an undiagnosed condition.

A tutor faced with a student in difficulty may, therefore, offer direct advise and/or onward referral. All interventions, however, should be followed up. Often, this will take the form of a simple email from the students stating that they have seen their personal tutor/GP/learning support as agreed.

> 'They (the tutors) were kind and listening and paying attention. I could take the first positive step after that. The interview itself is part of the intervention.' Third year student talking about the educational assessment interview.
>
> – taken from Evans and Brown (2009)

Outcomes

Clearly, academic support should never be targeted at helping students to pass exams, but should rather be targeted at helping them become competent doctors who pass exams along the way. It should be noted that successful completion of the course is not the only possible positive outcome for a student in difficulty. Students who discover that they do not wish to follow a career in medicine will benefit from transferring to another course, or may be able to leave carrying some academic credit with them. For students who are unable to reach the standards required of them on qualification, despite the help they receive in overcoming the issues facing them, failing to qualify should be seen as a positive outcome that protects patients (Box 17.3).

Issues

Communication with and within the medical school and clinical learning environment is important and students may need to be reassured that medical schools are supportive of students in difficulty, as some students may find this surprising.

Box 17.3 **Interventions**

Student A With encouragement, Adil started studying in the library at the end of the day before going home or to the bar. He spent two-thirds of his time reviewing topics and one-third of his time preparing topics that were likely to come up tomorrow, which he found highly rewarding. He experimented with different note taking techniques, and modified Cornell notes to ensure active learning whilst he was revising

Student B Richard started a learning diary to compare his hours of study with peers. He signed up for the student union chess and drama clubs. He started an 'OSCE' learning group with six other students and is now able to measure his depth and breadth of learning against others and discuss exams and the hidden curriculum with peers

Student C Elizabeth worked on strategies to give herself permission to be a learner, and found introducing herself to patients as 'only a medical student, just here to learn' was paradoxically empowering. She attended a course on 'how to learn clinical skills' and actively engaged with some peers in a clinical skills study group

Student D Tuan attended English conversation classes which boosted his confidence with English language. His personal tutor introduced him to a more patient-centred, holistic model for eliciting a patient history and went with him to the wards to practise history taking with patients and feedback. He was encouraged to join clubs, learn in a group and socialise with peers to build friendships and greater interpersonal skills. He also moved into medical student's halls

Student E Louise was referred to her GP and received treatment for her depression. She was followed-up to ensure that she was coping with her studies and through negotiation with her tutor she was allowed to repeat part of her third year. She progressed to fourth year with no apparent learning deficits

It may be important to consider the following:

- Liaising with other tutors/medical school/clinical supervisor so that information is shared and all are kept informed is important.
- Information should be logged in a central place to provide an overview and prevent duplication.
- Follow-up is important to prevent people slipping through the net.
- And finally, for the tutor working with students in difficulty, collaborating with colleagues, sharing problems or taking part in formal supervision is essential to prevent isolation and ensure a balanced view.

References

Brown J, Evans DE. Supporting students who struggle academically. *The newsletter of the Subject Centre for Medicine, Dentistry and Veterinary Medicine* 2005;01:1–8.

Dyrbye LN, Thomas MR, Shanafelt TD. Systematic review of depression, anxiety, and other indicators of psychological distress among U.S. and Canadian medical students. *Academic Medicine* 2006;81:354–373.

Evans D, Brown J. *How to Succeed at Medical School: An Essential Guide to Learning*. Oxford: Wiley-Blackwell, 2009.

Ford M, Masterton G, Cameron H, Kristmundsdottir F. Supporting struggling medical students. *Clinical Teacher* 2008;5(4):232–238.

Sayer M, Chaput de Saintonge M, Evans DE, Wood DF. Support for students with academic difficulties. *Medical Education* 2002;36:643–650.

Index

Note: page numbers in *italics* refer to figures, those in **bold** refer to tables and boxes

LIBRARY
EDUCATION CENTRE
PRINCESS ROYAL HOSPITAL